'Many women experience menopausal sy
treatments which can impact on their qualit
to support and guide those who may be str

'Women with cancer have for so long been left out of the menopause 'conversation'. Dani has worked tirelessly to support and advocate for the many women who suffer with menopause after cancer treatment and this is a hugely comprehensive summary of evidence-based information. As a menopause specialist, I will have no hesitation in recommending this to both the patients I see and the doctors who are looking after them.' **Dr Olivia Hum, GP and British Menopause Society Accredited Menopause Specialist**

'In my view, this is the much-awaited guide to navigating menopausal life post-cancer — it is an encyclopaedia and a compassionate hug all wrapped into one invaluable book. Dani has put all her collected knowledge and experience into one easy-to-read and supportive package!' **Dr Sarah Ball, GP and British Menopause Society Accredited Menopause Specialist**

'This straightforward, easy-to-understand book covers everything you need to know about how to manage menopause after cancer. Dani's personal experience, and her passion for supporting other people with similar experiences, have contributed to this brilliant resource to support you from surviving to thriving.' **Dr Claire Macaulay, Medical Oncologist (Breast), The Beatson West of Scotland Cancer Centre**

'Menopause symptoms have a huge impact on women's quality of life. Unfortunately, there is so much misinformation out there on how to manage these symptoms through diet and lifestyle — most of it is non-evidence-based nonsense! This book highlights evidence-based approaches to help women through their menopause and covers the latest science in this area. Dani, her book, and her organisation are a fantastic resource bringing together experience, evidence and compassion.' **Professor Sarah Berry, Department of Nutritional Sciences, King's College London and Chief Scientist at ZOE**

'This helpful guide presents multiple voices of women who have experienced the problems of menopause side by side with the opinions of medical experts and researchers in this difficult, and often controversial, area. Above all, Dani demonstrates the power of shared decision-making and the strength that people with cancer can gain from good information and support.' **Professor Richard Simcock, Consultant Oncologist and Macmillan Chief Medical Officer**

'Navigating Menopause After Cancer *is an urgently needed, deeply compassionate, and thoroughly evidence-based resource that fills a critical gap in caring for cancer survivors. As menopause specialists, we have witnessed firsthand how treatment-induced menopause can profoundly affect quality of life, yet remains under-discussed and under-treated in clinical settings. By bringing together leading experts across oncology, menopause care, nutrition and rehabilitation, this book offers not only information but also hope. It should be essential reading not just for survivors, but for every healthcare professional involved in cancer and menopause care.'* **Dr Susanne Hooper and Dr Melanie Hacking, GPs and British Menopause Society Accredited Menopause Specialists, Oxford Hormone Clinic**

'If you ever wanted to read one book on cancer and menopause — this is for you. Drawing from her own experience and that of many doctors and experts, Dani will guide you through the roller coaster hormonal journey that can follow cancer treatment and provide you with all the up-to-date information you need to navigate it successfully.' **Mr Vikram Talaulikar, Associate Specialist at the Reproductive Medicine, British Menopause Society Accredited Menopause Specialist**

'Early menopause after breast cancer treatment was like being kicked when I was down, and it's no exaggeration to say that Dani's work changed my life. Her dedication to helping women feel healthier,

happier and more in control, in a criminally under-researched area, has done the same for so many others. She writes with compassion, providing the information and support that should be available to women through their medical teams, but sadly isn't. This book should be prescribed to anyone emerging from cancer treatment having gone through early menopause.' **Rosamund Dean, Journalist and Author**

'As a breast cancer specialist nurse with many years of experience, I am truly grateful to be able to signpost those affected by breast cancer to Dani's book. It is an invaluable resource that offers both comfort and hope to individuals navigating life after a diagnosis. The book provides a wealth of knowledge that encourages women to engage in informed discussions with their healthcare teams and explore the options available to them as they manage menopausal symptoms.'
Jackie Wright, Clinical Nurse Specialist, Future Dreams House

'For anyone diagnosed with cancer and thrown into menopause — this book is a must-read. Most oncologists and surgeons are not menopause specialists, and most GPs are not cancer specialists. Women have historically fallen through the cracks, and it's left them in a cancer no-man's land. Fortunately, this huge unmet need is becoming more and more recognised and help is now out there. This book, and the Menopause and Cancer organisation, are a fabulous place to start!' **Dr Alison Macbeth, GP and British Menopause Society Accredited Menopause Specialist**

'Love this book! As a nutritionist who practises in both the oncology and menopause care worlds, I see firsthand how desperate women are for evidence-based information that empowers them to feel they can manage this sometimes abrupt transition into menopause — often years before it would naturally occur. Dani does a masterful job of delivering valuable information that can replace the overabundance of often confusing online information with credible advice and help women feel they aren't alone in their struggles.'
Hillary Wright, Registered Dietitian, Senior Nutritionist at the Dana-Farber Cancer Institute

NAVIGATING MENOPAUSE AFTER CANCER

NAVIGATING **MENOPAUSE** AFTER **CANCER**

A comprehensive, empowering guide
to all your treatment options,
where to get help and how to feel better

DANI BINNINGTON

Editor: Imogen Fortes | Copy editor: Jaqui Lewis | Cover design: Laura Woussen – www.laurawoussen.co.uk, @laurawoussendesign

For more information, email hello@healthywholeme.com

ISBN: 978-1-0684999-0-6

GET YOUR FREE GIFT!

To make this book as practical as possible, I've created a digital handbook to accompany it. This handbook includes links to other organisations, helpful tips and resources, and even studies you can share with your doctors.

Simply scan the QR code below – leave your email and we'll send the handbook straight to your inbox.

You can also get a copy by visiting:

www.menopauseandcancer.org/book

DEDICATION

This book is dedicated to the women in my family we have lost to cancer, whose strength and love continue to guide me. It is written for the generations to come, so they may face life with knowledge and hope.

To my daughters, you are my heart, my everything and my reason to keep going. You are the future of women's health and it is bright!

And to all my fellow survivors, this is for you: a guide of knowledge, a testament to our resilience, struggles and our shared journey towards healing. Your journey is unique. I see you.

Contents

INTRODUCTION

If you are reading this book, the chances are that you too have had a cancer diagnosis and now find yourself dealing with menopause symptoms. I have met many people who say that menopause after cancer is harder than chemotherapy, radiotherapy and surgery all together.

This book is for you.

Although menopause discussions have surged in the UK in recent years, with the US catching on more recently, women with a history of cancer have felt largely excluded from the conversation. In the UK, doctors, celebrities and what felt like an army of women have taken to social media, TV and the press to educate others and share their experiences. Women were becoming increasingly vocal about the profound impact that perimenopause and menopause can have on one's life. There was a collective 'aha' moment and, soon, everyone was talking about treatment options, such as hormone replacement therapy (HRT). Alongside this, a genuine sense of solidarity emerged. Women had been ignored by science and medicine for far too long! Misreporting of data had led to inadequate treatment options for symptoms like sleepless nights, anxiety, hot flushes, itchy skin, dry vagina, loss of libido and many other life-impacting issues. When it was revealed that many doctors had received no mandatory menopause training – even though every second patient is a woman – all hell broke loose. A much-needed 'menopause revolution' was under way. It felt as though we had finally understood: women deserve to feel well, age in good health and have their needs met.

But while passionate campaigners gathered outside Britain's Houses of Parliament, I couldn't help but think, 'What about me?' What about us? What about women with a history of cancer?

This book is here to answer that question and provide support and guidance to cancer survivors facing menopause – because, frankly, no one was talking about us.

When preparing for my own surgical menopause after breast cancer, I searched everywhere and could hardly find any information specific to cancer survivors. It was as if we had been forgotten in this conversation. While HRT was on everyone's lips, all I could find were statements that it was contraindicated for women with a history of cancer. I was confused, then I became outraged. Outraged that no one seemed to be asking the tough questions or acknowledging the unique challenges cancer survivors face when navigating menopause. I was angry that the information and support we desperately needed were almost entirely non-existent.

This outrage quickly turned into a mission. I became obsessed with finding out what options were out there and how we, as a community, could do better – not just for cancer survivors like me but for *anyone* after *any* type of cancer.

I want to ensure that this 'menopause revolution' reaches everyone. To me, this means being truly inclusive of all women – regardless of how they choose to manage menopause, where they come from, or their personal and health histories. And it's about including everyone who has ovaries in this conversation – whether they identify as women or not. While I often use the term 'women', because many studies I will reference have been done on females, this book's purpose is to reach everyone who experiences menopause after cancer.

My Story

I was 33 and a mum to three young girls when I found a lump in my left breast. Our twin girls were two and my eldest daughter was four and there was no way we could have foreseen that this lump would change the course of our lives for ever. But it did. Diagnosed with a triple-negative, highly aggressive tumour, I embarked on active cancer treatment. Like so many of you reading this, I stepped onto an escalator on which each step pulled us further along an unknown path. At first, I was too scared to ask any questions. I did as I was told and as a family we did our best to get through our ordeal. My world as I had known it had changed for ever and all I desperately wanted was to see my little girls start school.

Today, as I am writing this, I have teenage girls in secondary school and college and I can't express how deeply grateful I am. I know I had luck on my side.

During chemotherapy my periods stopped, and, although I was told this could happen because of the cancer treatment, no one mentioned that it was actually putting me into temporary menopause. When my periods returned a few months after I finished chemotherapy, I thought that would be the end of it and I could just get on with the rest of my life.

But once my active cancer treatment was 'over', and everyone around me had congratulated me on 'being done', that was when I started to crumble. I had no idea – initially – how to rebuild my house and life. I thought I just needed to recover physically, so I changed my diet, started running, and believed that, by being a much healthier version of myself, I'd stand a better chance of surviving. Looking back, I know none of the drastic changes I made were necessary. They gave me a sense of control and hope, yet my mental health was still at an all-time low. It wasn't until my mum encouraged me to seek counselling and my mother-in-law ushered me to my first yoga class that I began to find some relief mentally. During yoga, I felt a little less anxious, more present; counselling allowed me some space to process what had happened to us.

I also learned that I carry the BRCA1 gene mutation, which added more concern and worry as this increases the risks of ovarian cancer and more breast cancers, and led me to make more difficult decisions. But with the tools I had gathered by then – yoga, therapy, diet, complementary strategies and community – I felt empowered to make those decisions with a little more confidence. All these changes helped me feel more hopeful about my future and more in control of my recovery. While my wonderful doctors gave me the cancer treatments and medical support I needed, I soon realised that I could become an active participant in my recovery and healing. And that, in itself, was empowering. I became more hopeful for a future. I felt I was clawing back some of the control that cancer wiped away.

My challenges when navigating surgical menopause

Two years after my initial cancer diagnosis, I opted to have a double mastectomy to reduce my risk of more breast cancers. Two years after that, I had my Fallopian tubes surgically removed, which reduced my risk of ovarian cancer by a large proportion – but not completely – and so another two years later, at the age of 39, I took the plunge and opted to have my ovaries removed, to do everything I could to reduce my risks of ovarian cancer. We have lost all the women on my dad's side of the family to this disease and so it was the right thing for me to do. This was the beginning of a new journey for me and the reason I am here writing this book.

As I prepared for the removal of my ovaries, I found a big contrast to the discussions I'd had around my double mastectomy. When I planned for that, I was given numerous options – whether to go flat, whether to have a reconstruction, whether to keep my nipples or not. I had discussions with my doctors and I was actively involved in making choices. But when it came to the bilateral oophorectomy (the removal of both my ovaries), there was no talk of what life would be like post surgery. There were no discussions around how early menopause might affect me or how I could manage the transition. Some doctors said, 'Let's wait and see how you do,' others said I could opt for hormone replacement therapy, while others ruled it out completely. Some warned me of the impact of early menopause on my heart, brain and bone health, but offered no solutions. It felt very doom and gloom, and whichever way I looked I felt I couldn't win.

But I'm lucky to have had the support to advocate for myself, to have family who encouraged me to seek second opinions. I asked countless questions until I fully understood what my options were to manage surgical menopause after my specific type of breast cancer. By the time I walked into surgery, I was empowered by knowledge. I understood what my doctors could do for me, and what I could do for myself.

Creating Community and Change

Between my own diagnosis over twelve years ago and today lies a long journey of personal transformation. Initially, when I tried to figure out how I was best going to manage menopause for myself, I set up my first private Facebook group. I was hoping to ask others to share with me what they knew. What happened next was astonishing: within weeks hundreds of women had joined, and soon it was thousands. These were people from all corners of the world, each with a different cancer diagnosis, but all facing similar struggles. They echoed my experiences: they didn't know where to turn, they were overwhelmed by debilitating symptoms, and many had no idea menopause was even going to be happening to them, let alone become such a big problem. And so I realised that there was this huge void.

At that time, I was already working in the wellbeing industry as a yoga teacher and organising workshops and webinars on different wellbeing topics. It seemed natural to take my next step: to search for and invite doctors and other experts with specialist experience who could help educate the members of our menopause and cancer Facebook community. And so I began facilitating workshops – connecting a growing network of experts with our growing community of women.

Later, I curated the Empowered Menopause After Cancer programme, where, alongside the experts, I helped guide women through actionable steps to feel better. It was – and still is – a real privilege to be a small part of these women's journeys, helping them figure out what their options are and to regain some sense of control and hope.

This led me to co-curate the UK's first programme for young adults with cancer in collaboration with the charity Trekstock. This initiative was recognised with a prestigious charity award for its impact, and I went on to deliver workshops for other organisations. Yet I knew this still wasn't helping enough people.

In the summer of 2022, nine years after my cancer diagnosis, I found myself sitting on the sofa of *This Morning*, a UK TV breakfast show, to speak about my experience. It was there that I announced the launch of The Menopause and Cancer Podcast. Since then, every single Wednesday I have released a new episode in which I interview the most incredible medical experts and survivors. The podcast provides evidence-based information and practical tips, and reaches hundreds of thousands of people all over the world. Doctors and charities now recommend it to their patients, and the feedback I've received has been both humbling and motivating to keep going. These podcast conversations have led to hundreds of women reaching out to me, telling me their stories and struggles.

And so I knew: we needed to do better. In 2022, I founded Menopause and Cancer, the world's only not-for-profit organisation dedicated to supporting this unique community – our community.

As an organisation, we bring together thought-leading experts to educate both survivors and healthcare professionals, in order to try to bring about the change that is so desperately needed. We have created a movement, we are hosting a global conversation. We're raising awareness of what it's like to be a patient with this very specific set of circumstances. We're getting all parties involved listening to one another and we're all learning. It is these experts' knowledge and information, alongside my own learnings and those of our community, that I want to share in this book.

Today, I receive numerous messages from people every week who say our work has transformed their lives for the better. They tell me they've learned more in one of our workshops than in years of navigating survivorship on their own. They no longer feel isolated – they know there's a whole community out there that truly 'gets it'. It's an honour and a privilege to be part of this journey, to meet with so many wonderful people, and now I'm so grateful to share a part of your journey with you too.

'No one ever said that my cancer treatment would make me menopausal!'

'My chemically induced menopause is making my life pure misery, my joint pain and body aches are so bad I feel about 90, when I'm half that age.'

'I was refused HRT but was not given any other options.'

Menopause symptoms vary greatly from one person to the next; your personal values and circumstances will play a role in how you manage things too.[1] Whether your menopause is temporary or permanent, due to chemotherapy, surgery, radiotherapy or hormone therapy, you are not alone. This book is here to support you.

If your experience is similar to that of many people in our community, then you too may feel isolated, not knowing who in your medical team can help you. Or you are confused about your treatment options and might feel you've not had the help you need. Each of your experiences is different, but one thing I know: by the time you are reading this, you have been through so much!

Cancer alone is a huge life shock. Menopause is an additional and enormous change for our bodies, impacting us physically, mentally and emotionally. If it happens as a result of cancer treatment, it feels like the insult to your injury. And yet it's the unexpected, long-term side effect that no one is talking about. It is no wonder we have hundreds of thousands of cancer survivors thinking that putting up with their menopause symptoms is the only choice they have.

But know that you have options too, and you are not alone. Globally, over 9 million women are diagnosed with cancer each year.[2] It's a number that continues to rise. Alarmingly, cancer rates are increasing not only overall but also among younger women. While advances in treatment mean that more women are surviving cancer than ever before, many are left navigating the long-term effects of their treatment, including the challenges of menopause.

'I don't really want to complain as I am so grateful for having survived cancer, but I'm really struggling.'

'I am fed up with everyone talking about how brilliant HRT is but I can't take it!'

'No one mentioned the immediate onset of menopause before my hysterectomy.'

Managing menopause after a cancer diagnosis requires a multifaceted approach. It's essential to do your research, ask questions and – currently – advocate for yourself. By raising awareness of this global issue, we can work together to ensure that women everywhere receive the support and care they need to thrive.

In the following chapters, I'll walk you through all of your treatment options, share some personal strategies, and show you what I wish I'd known when navigating this challenging journey. You'll hear from experts and other cancer survivors, and you'll be empowered to take control of your next steps. Healing is three-dimensional and often surprising – you never know what might make a difference.

After reading this book, you will:

- Understand ALL your treatment options (medical, hormonal, non-hormonal and complementary therapies).
- Understand how you can support yourself daily (through diet, movement and a host of other lifestyle choices).
- Be able to craft your own action plan so that you can become actively involved in the decisions behind your treatments.

This is a process, and going through it will mean that each one of you will take something different from this book. Some things will be highly relevant to you, others less so, at least for now. But know, you are not alone – we are all out there and we've got your back.

Whatever your cancer.

Whatever stage you're at.

Whichever way you arrived at menopause.

Regardless of your age, ethnicity or background.

Whether you identify as a woman or not.

This book is for you.

This book is your guide to taking back control. Let's start this journey together.

CHAPTER 1
WHY IS MENOPAUSE AFTER CANCER DIFFERENT?

Menopause, a natural phase marking the end of a woman's reproductive years, can be a challenging transition on its own. But when cancer treatments intervene, triggering menopause prematurely, or meaning that your menopause treatment options differ from those of a woman without of a history of cancer, the impact on your current and future physical, mental and emotional health can be huge.[3]

Women whose menopause is induced by cancer treatment often experience more severe and complex symptoms compared to those who go through natural menopause. The combination of sudden hormonal changes, the effects of cancer treatments and medication itself, and in many cases limited treatment options for symptom management contribute to this increased severity. And of course, the psychological impact of a cancer diagnosis, combined with abrupt menopause, can heighten feelings of anxiety and uncertainty. It's hard to say what someone might experience, but symptoms range from physical to emotional to mental, and many women experience a whole array of them.[4]

This chapter delves into your cancer-induced menopause and helps you understand how you got here and what your next steps could look like. I want to acknowledge that if you are struggling – that's normal.

What you're experiencing is real, it's not just in your head, it's okay to need support – and you are not alone. I know you might want to get straight into finding solutions to help you feel better and manage your menopause symptoms. I've been there too, just wanting the answers. But understanding the basics of what's happening in your body is a crucial first step. I had no idea what was happening to me when I went through it. Take your time – we're on this journey together now; you've made your next step by reading this book.

Understanding Menopause

Menopause marks the end of a woman's menstrual cycle and is characterised by a decline in oestrogen and progesterone production, which can lead to various physical and emotional symptoms. Hot flushes, anxiety, night sweats, vaginal dryness, mood swings and sleep disturbances are just some of the most common symptoms. Menopause is diagnosed in retrospect, once you have not had any periods for 12 months.

Natural menopause occurs as a result of ageing. Medically induced menopause can be triggered by cancer treatments like chemotherapy, surgery to remove ovaries, anti-hormone treatment or radiation therapy to the pelvis. It can happen at any age.

Understanding the differences between these two types of menopause is so important for effective management and support, and that's what we're going to be addressing throughout this book. Every day I hear the stories of countless women who say they were not prepared for the menopause that followed their cancer treatment, and some even feel like menopause after cancer was like sinking into a big black hole. But I'm here to show you there is light at the end of the tunnel.

Research and science have failed to adequately address the impact cancer treatments have on ovarian function and hence on cancer survivors as a whole.[5] And while this may seem bleak, I am confident that the landscape will transform.

To begin, let's reflect a little on your journey so far to understand what has happened and how you arrived at this point, and acknowledge where you are now. From there, we will identify your goals and create a vision for your future, allowing you to craft your action plan. As you journey through this book, I will introduce you to many doctors and experts who have shared their expertise with me and our community over the years. One such expert is Mr Vikram Talaulikar. As an associate specialist at the Reproductive Medicine Unit at University College London Hospitals NHS Foundation Trust, Mr Talaulikar has spent years working with cancer patients dealing with treatment-induced menopause. His extensive knowledge and his encouragement of me have been invaluable in shaping this book.

How Cancer Treatments Trigger Menopause

Cancer treatments can disrupt the delicate hormonal balance in the body, leading to premature or immediate menopause in individuals undergoing therapy.

Surgery

Did you have surgery in which your ovaries were removed? Procedures such as a bilateral oophorectomy, the surgical removal of both functioning ovaries, can abruptly stop oestrogen and progesterone production. Since these hormones play a central role in regulating the menstrual cycle, their sudden absence results in an immediate onset of permanent menopause. Women undergoing oophorectomy often experience intense menopausal symptoms within hours due to the sudden profound hormonal changes. Mr Vikram Talaulikar explains: 'The gradual withdrawal of hormones that happens with natural perimenopause followed by menopause allows women to adapt to the changing hormones over time to an extent, but this does not happen with abrupt surgical menopause. If you have had a hysterectomy and your ovaries were also removed, this would have also plunged you into surgical menopause.'

> *'I had a full hysterectomy to help treat bowel cancer. I wasn't prepared for the extreme symptoms of surgical menopause. At 44, I had perimenopause symptoms prior to my surgery but mild. About three weeks after surgery the nights sweats, hair loss and skin changes kicked in! Hormonal shock was something my doctor mentioned and it can be worse in some women than others. My hair fell out in handfuls, and the hot flushes – omg! It's a rough ride.'* **Georgina**

Chemotherapy

Certain chemotherapeutic agents can damage the ovarian follicles responsible for hormone production. This damage can lead to a decline in ovarian function, resulting in temporary or permanent menopause. The severity and length of menopausal symptoms experienced during chemotherapy can vary depending on factors such as age and the type and dosage of chemotherapy drugs given. Your periods may stop temporarily during chemotherapy or they may stop for good. Doctors don't really know if they will come back and the uncertainty can be tough to sit with. The older you are, the higher the risk that this menopause will be permanent. Mr Vikram Talaulikar explains: 'With chemotherapy, you can go quickly into the menopause. This is because chemotherapy drugs are designed to seek and destroy dividing cells and do not differentiate between cancer cells and the follicles containing a woman's eggs (oocytes), which are also very active. As a result, many of these are also destroyed during treatment.' He adds, 'For younger women who have a huge number of eggs remaining and only have mild chemotherapy – their store will reduce. But for a woman in her late thirties, chemotherapy will most likely wipe out her store of eggs.'

> *'I feel frustrated at the absence of a full conversation about the menopause and symptoms. I appreciate that when you're first diagnosed, it's hard to do anything but just get by. However, I wish there'd been a more open conversation during and after about the emotional and physical impact of chemotherapy and going into menopause. I also had Zoladex injections to switch my ovaries off at the same time – in hindsight that was huge. Things like vaginal dryness were not mentioned, and the impact on sex life. Fairly soon after chemo, I had to go for a smear test – I was so nervous – the nurse was brilliant and aware of potential discomfort. The nurse commented that the system appears to be more proactive in communicating to men the impact on sex life (of some cancer treatments) than to women. Emotionally, the fallout of menopause and cancer treatment has been huge for me.'* **Ali**

Radiation therapy

Pelvic radiation therapy, commonly used in the treatment of gynaecological and colorectal cancers, can inadvertently affect ovarian function by exposing the ovaries to radiation. Radiation can cause direct DNA damage to ovarian follicles, and this can reduce ovarian reserves, leading to a decline in hormone production and egg activity, and therefore menopause symptoms. The extent of ovarian damage and the likelihood of menopause depends on factors such as age, the radiation dose and how close the ovaries are to the treatment area.

'It's difficult to say what caused my symptoms. I was already menopausal before my cancer diagnosis. Radiotherapy in itself wasn't too challenging for me, but all my menopause symptoms became so much worse all of a sudden.' **Susanne**

Hormone (endocrine) therapy

Some cancer treatments, particularly those aimed at hormone-sensitive cancers, involve therapies that block or suppress hormone production. For example, anti-oestrogen therapies such as tamoxifen, aromatase inhibitors and medicines to switch off ovaries are commonly used in breast cancer treatment. Endocrine treatment puts you into chemical menopause or gives you side effects that mimic those of menopause, and it is often prescribed for up to five to ten years. On top of that, many of these medications come with their own side effects, which can be very tough to manage. Mr Talaulikar says, 'Endocrine therapies can cause severe menopause symptoms and have a profound impact on quality of life.'

'Menopause was NOT mentioned when I was being told which drugs I'd be given. The hot flushes and other side effects kicked in quickly. I started on letrozole, which was horrendous – insomnia, fast weight gain, worse hot flushes, no libido, dry skin and extreme aches in all my joints where I felt like I was trapped in a 90-year-old body. Mentally that was the worst part as I

couldn't move easily and enjoy walks beforehand, which had really helped me through chemo. My knees and ankles were the worst. However, listening to Dani's podcast I learned there are other options, so I talked to my oncologist and had a break for six weeks, in which time I felt so much better! After my oncologist swapped me to other drugs and again, I learned through the podcast and the Facebook group to try different brands to see which ones have better/worse side effects for me. Now I feel much better (even if all the local pharmacies are sick of me ringing around looking for the brand I want!). I'm at a stage now (just over two years from starting the meds) where I feel more comfortable and things seem to be settling a bit.' **Hannah**

A Complex Menopause

Regardless of the type of cancer treatment you've undergone, experiencing menopause symptoms is often complex and can be overwhelming, and requires careful management.

When ovarian function re-establishes itself after cancer treatment, it can mean that you later go through perimenopause and menopause again. The younger the individual when they receive treatments such as chemotherapy, the higher the chances that ovarian function (periods/ovulation) will resume after a few months or years of temporary menopause following completion of the cancer treatment.

Perhaps your secondary cancer diagnosis required new treatment protocols that induced or will induce menopause?

Or were you told to stop your HRT (hormone replacement therapy) as soon as you were told you had cancer? Having to come off HRT, on top of their cancer diagnosis, might feel like a big loss to many.[6]

'I was told to stop my HRT immediately after I was diagnosed with breast cancer and it was terrifying. HRT had been such a lifeline for me. I'd finally started feeling like myself again after years of struggling with menopause symptoms. The thought of losing that support felt overwhelming and I worried more about stopping the HRT than my cancer treatment I was about to start. What made it even worse was the complete lack of support. I was just told to stop. I felt completely alone in navigating this huge change and so I had no choice but to go cold turkey. When I tried to ask for help, I felt dismissed, like it wasn't a big deal or a priority. But for me, it was a big deal and it was scary.' **Helena**

You're in transition

Having to deal with everything your cancer diagnosis brings with it is a huge upheaval, but discovering that you are also in menopause, or that your cancer treatment may give you menopause symptoms, can be hugely overwhelming. In a recent study 80–93% of the people surveyed felt somewhat, very or completely uninvolved in their menopause-related treatment decisions.[7]

It's also a very confusing time because symptoms of menopause and cancer-treatment side effects can look very similar, so you are constantly asking yourself, which are cancer-related symptoms and what is menopause? Is it still chemo brain, or menopausal brain fog? Are you suffering from anxiety because you've been diagnosed with cancer or is it anxiety because of your low hormone levels? Maybe a bit of both? You probably have more questions than answers. You're in transition.

And while trying to work out how to navigate the challenges of menopause, you might also be looking for 'your old self' again, the 'pre-cancer you'. If you're anything like I was, then you'll be acutely aware that the 'old you' is gone, but you haven't found the 'new you' yet. A wonderful lady named Dawn, who enrolled in my empowered menopause programme a few years back, sent me this quote: 'I am at that awkward stage where my old self is gone but my new self hasn't fully been born.' This sums up beautifully how I felt.

I felt as though I lost myself for a long time after my cancer diagnosis. The carefree Dani was replaced by a Dani consumed with worry that my cancer would return with a vengeance. Every ache and pain led me to catastrophise – the 'what ifs' were a constant threat. Even long after everyone around me had celebrated the end of my active treatment, I still found myself unable to do so. I realised my 'new normal' was nothing like I expected. I had changed and it hit me hard.

In response, I created significant life changes for myself. I threw myself into eating healthily and I almost became a bit obsessed with eating differently than before cancer, but it also taught me how to cook, especially with vegetables and fresh whole foods. After a lot of trial and error, I became a good cook. Actively taking part in my recovery and healing gave me hope – hope that I was on the right track and a glimmer of belief that I might be able to do this.

It was also at this point that my mother-in-law sent me off to my first yoga class. Although my first few months on the mat were filled with worries that my wig would slip off, I found enormous relief from anxiety while practising yoga. I got hooked and eventually became a yoga teacher myself. But I never felt that what I was doing was enough. I stopped drinking alcohol, removed all toxic household products, went to counselling, hypnotherapy, sound workshops, tried mistletoe therapy, IV infusions – you name it. I didn't leave a stone unturned in my quest to feel better emotionally, physically and mentally and to keep cancer at bay.

These massive lifestyle and behaviour changes meant I was transforming as a person. Even socialising was different; going to parties and dinners as a sober person was different. That alone was a huge adjustment. I was no longer dancing on tables at 3am; instead I was sneaking away way before midnight.

What I didn't realise then was that I was already in transition. By creating this new version of myself, I was letting go of parts of the old me. Month by month, year by year, I was changing. Without realising it, I was slowly becoming the 'new me', the new version of post-cancer Dani. I was creating her, I just did not know it at the time.

If I could go back now, I would wrap my younger self in my arms and tell her how incredible she is for her huge effort, for showing up and giving it her all. I would also tell her that it's okay simply to be sometimes: to take a deep breath, relax her shoulders and share some of the burdens she carried so heavily each day.

And I wonder if you too feel you are in transition somehow? Have you changed since your diagnosis?

This time of transition is also a time for mourning: mourning the life we had before cancer, for who we were, perhaps for how our bodies used to look, and of course the mourning for our dreams, the knowledge that our future might be very different to what we anticipated it would be. And I feel that it's important to acknowledge and then to mourn that loss. I really miss that carefree version of me.

Many of you reading this will also be confronted with the loss of your dream of a family, even if you had never really decided whether you wanted to become a biological parent or not. This can weigh heavily;

the sadness of having to let go of our dreams can feel too much at times. The loss of fertility is for many the hardest part of their cancer diagnosis.

I believe that after a life shock your life can never go back to normal, because the experience deeply transforms your perspective and priorities. These changes become a part of you, reshaping your identity and how you move forward. Once we truly understand this, we can take part in this process and discover what it might look like. Once we've shed, let go and mourned, we can make space for something new. Let's do that together!

A Time for Discovery

Sometimes, you might feel lost, unsure of whether you are coming or going. I know that some days I wake up feeling immense gratitude to be alive, while simultaneously fearing for my life. Being in this transition phase gives us a key opportunity to explore new possibilities. Yes, I will go into much detail about what is in your menopause after cancer toolkit to help you with your symptoms and also help you look after your long-term health, but I think it's so important that we also address the bigger picture. That there is so much that changes in your life on top of the many menopause symptoms you may be experiencing. And that therefore, of course, it can be so tough.

Ask yourself: What gives me joy now? I had to redefine that for myself because what used to bring me joy no longer did. I needed to find new ways of exercising appropriately for my new post-surgery body and to seek out new hobbies and ways to connect with friends.

I think we all need to be bold and brave and dream BIG. Envisage how you want to feel and create a vision of who you want to become. Paint this new person really clearly in your mind: what does the new you do? What does the new you look like? How does the new you feel?

Understand that you have total agency over this process. You can set your intentions so that the 'new you' is who you truly want to be. Alongside finding solutions to your symptoms, you can address the 'bigger picture' and actively shape your post-cancer diagnosis life.

Reflections and Positive Actions

Reflection exercises are a really helpful way to understand and digest each chapter, and figure out if the information is relevant to you right now and whether you want to take action. Your experience is unique to you and these exercises will help you connect with your own needs, values and goals. By reflecting on your physical, emotional and mental wellbeing and by acknowledging what has happened to you, you can better understand which areas of your life need attention. Throughout the book I will be suggesting that you set aside some time to complete your own reflections. Consider them your mini-moments of mindfulness. They're your opportunities to pause and think for a moment, allowing you to address all aspects of your wellbeing. This is the practical bit. This is where you translate what you have read into what matters in your own life. This is when you become more than the reader. This is when you take action and are well on your way to becoming the empowered patient. It's no good knowing all the facts without doing something about it, so please do take some time out to work through the exercises.

You can either write down your answers in a journal or take some time to think through them carefully. And remember to download your digital handbook (the QR code is in the front of the book) as I have added helpful links and tips for you to go alongside this book.

REFLECTIONS

Take a few moments to reflect...

1. How did you arrive in menopause after cancer?
2. Did you know it was going to happen in that way?
3. Have you changed since your diagnosis?
4. Do you mourn your pre-cancer self?
5. What do you want your new you to become?

POSITIVE ACTIONS

1. What can you do for yourself today that makes you feel good? Take a bath, enjoy a walk, phone a friend.
2. Write down three things you want to add to your life that will bring you joy and support your transition.
3. Download the digital handbook to support your process while reading this book.

CHAPTER 2
YOUR MENOPAUSE SYMPTOMS

If you are recovering from surgery, radiotherapy or chemotherapy, it can be incredibly challenging to untangle which symptoms are due to your cancer treatment and which are menopause-related from lack of hormones. If you are on an endocrine treatment, like tamoxifen or aromatase inhibitors, the side effects of these medications can complicate things further. Joint pain, fatigue and anxiety, for example, can be consequences of both cancer treatment and menopause, making it very confusing to figure out what's what.

Before you can even begin to address your symptoms, let's identify exactly what you are experiencing, how often and to what severity. By getting a clear overview of your symptoms, you can better understand your needs and develop a tailored approach to improve your quality of life.

At many of our workshops, I go through the symptoms associated with menopause, and I'm always amazed at how often someone has a lightbulb moment and exclaims, 'I had no idea this was a symptom of menopause!' It's a relief for them because understanding that a symptom is menopause-related can provide reassurance, allowing them to address it with the right knowledge and resources, rather than feeling confused or worried that the symptom they're experiencing is related to their cancer.

You might already track your symptoms but, if you don't, it's really important that you start doing so now. Each time you take stock of what you are experiencing can be a new discovery, because for many people symptoms really do fluctuate and their severity can come and go in waves. You might not be doing anything differently, but you may have phases when you are so wiped of energy that you suddenly have no idea how you will get to the end of the day, or have no energy for your usual workout routine. And then all of a sudden things start to flow much better, again for no obvious reason. Know that this is normal and adapt your days slightly.

Tracking your symptoms, which I call your 'check in with yourself session', will help you:

- Communicate more effectively with your healthcare professionals to ensure you get the most out of your appointments.

- Recognise when a strategy is working: improvements in symptoms might be subtle at first, so having a baseline for comparison helps you understand what is working and what isn't.

Ideally, you should track your symptoms regularly – every few weeks. We have a symptom checklist in the Resources section on the Menopause and Cancer website (www.menopauseandcancer.org) and I have linked it in the digital handbook for you. But you can also simply use a notepad and pen or your journal.

Which Symptoms Are You Currently Experiencing?

Your symptoms may all be bothering you, or you may have one in particular that is causing problems. When you track your symptoms it is helpful to be as detailed as you can be as this will help your doctor in determining what treatment might work best for you. For example, if you write down joint pain, ask yourself:

- Can you remember when it started?
- Do your joints ache all day long, or is it worse first thing in the morning?
- Does the pain improve after a walk?
- How bad is it on a scale from 1–10?
- If you're on long-term anti-hormone medication, did your joint pain start with the medication, or have you had it before?

Menopause after cancer comes with a long list of potential symptoms (see pages 30–32). While everyone's experience is different, you might find that many of them feel all too familiar.

Go through your symptom checker methodically. Find a clear, quiet 15 minutes for yourself and take stock of the symptoms you're experiencing. What is important is that you become crystal clear about what you are experiencing at the moment. There's no value in comparing yourself to anyone else; it doesn't matter if it seems like others are experiencing more severe symptoms or appear to be sailing through it all with ease. Your journey is unique, and it's important to focus on just yourself. There will always be someone worse off or better off than you.

At this point, I'd like to introduce you to another expert whose unwavering support for our cancer community has been instrumental in shaping this book. Dr Alison Macbeth is a renowned expert in supporting breast cancer patients navigating the challenges of menopause symptoms.

> *I am an NHS breast surgical speciality doctor, a women's health GP, and a British Menopause Society accredited menopause specialist who specialises in menopause after breast cancer.*
>
> *I was inspired to start a menopause clinic within my NHS breast unit after seeing patients who were suffering greatly with menopause symptoms after cancer. It is such an unmet need, as most breast surgeons and oncologists are not menopause trained, and indeed most menopause specialists are not breast trained, so there was such a void in resources and treatment for these women. I believe all women, including those treated for cancer, deserve access to high-quality, evidence-based menopause care and treatment. Every woman should be empowered to seek help and support at every stage of their treatment, and be treated as a whole person and not 'just a set of boobs'.*
>
> *While Dani was writing this book and I was helping to review and edit some chapters, I went for a routine NHS breast screening. Unfortunately, I was diagnosed with lobular breast cancer. I had been on HRT for a few years, to treat menopause symptoms but also mainly for bone protection as every single female member of my family has early-onset osteoporosis. As my cancer was oestrogen receptor-positive, I had to wean myself off and*

eventually stop HRT. After surgery, I started on an aromatase inhibitor, which reduces my risk of breast cancer recurrence. Some women tolerate these well, but the majority of women do struggle with the side effects. Aromatase inhibitors reduce your oestrogen to negligible levels, and thus side effects to expect are joint pains and stiffness, muscle tightness and stiffness, hot and cold flushes and sweats, insomnia, low mood, low libido, brain fog and very frequently genito-urinary syndrome of menopause, which includes urinary frequency and urgency, vaginal and vulval dryness and burning, painful sex, and increased risk of urine infections. In a lot of women, however, these side effects can settle over time, especially the joint pains.

Personally, I have struggled with muscle stiffness, making it difficult for me to run, insomnia, sweats and flushes, brain fog, low mood and urinary frequency. This might also be a consequence of stopping my systemic HRT. Acne was an unpleasant side effect of letrozole and just felt like 'another kick in the teeth'!

All women will have a different menopause experience, and everyone has different symptoms at different times. What you are struggling with now may be different to your symptoms in the next 6 to 12 months. As a menopause expert helping cancer patients, I've always strived to understand and support my patients, to see their struggles and needs. But now, after my own breast cancer diagnosis, I find myself in their shoes. This journey has given me an even deeper understanding – one I never expected. I now experience what so many of you experience too on every level, and it has brought a new perspective to my work. I am even more determined to offer support, hope, guidance and compassion, knowing first-hand just how vital it is.

Your Symptom Checker

Symptom	Not at all	A little	A lot	Comments
Fatigue, lack of energy				
Poor sleep, insomnia				
Anxiety				
Low mood				
Depression				
Irritability				
Brain fog, difficulty concentrating				
Panic attacks				
Feeling faint/dizzy				
Pins and needles, crawling ants under skin feeling				
Headaches				
Heart palpitations				

Symptom	Not at all	A little	A lot	Comments
Loss of sex drive, low or no libido				
Low self-esteem				
Difficulty concentrating				
Hot flushes				
Cold flushes				
Night sweats				
Changes in body odour				
Increased food sensitivities/ allergies				
Digestive issues/ bloating/ heartburn/ constipation				
Weight gain				
Hair changes/ thinning				

Symptom	Not at all	A little	A lot	Comments
Skin changes/ dryness/ itching/acne				
Dry eyes/ brittle nails				
Oral health changes				
Burning mouth syndrome				
Tinnitus				
Muscle and joint pain				
Restless legs				

Check your bits down below

Sure, discussing issues 'down below' or a loss of libido can be uncomfortable, but doctors need specific information about what is burning, stinging or bleeding to treat symptoms correctly. A few years ago I had no idea what was what, and had to embark on a learning journey about sexual health. I was in my forties when I got a mirror out for the first time to have a good look at my genitals. Menopause experts encourage us to do so. When explaining my new knowledge of appropriately naming our 'bits' to my kids, I said, 'There is an "IN" in "vagINa", so you know it's on the inside. Your vulva is on the outside.' They, of course, rolled their eyes!

All joking aside, it is in fact crucial to use the correct names for our anatomy to improve communication with doctors and receive the right treatment. This is why I've put genito-urinary symptoms in a separate section from other menopause symptoms. The loss of oestrogen can affect multiple organs and tissues in the genital and urinary systems and lead to vaginal and vulval issues, and can also affect the bladder and urethra, as well as the pelvic floor. Collectively, these symptoms are known as the genito-urinary syndrome of menopause (GSM).[8] This syndrome can significantly affect the vulva (the outside genitals), leading to symptoms such as dryness, thinning of the skin, irritation, burning and increased sensitivity. The skin of the vulva can become more fragile, making it prone to tearing or discomfort, especially during activities like sex, exercise or even wearing tight clothing. Symptoms also include vaginal dryness, irritation, pain and burning, painful intercourse, shrinking of the labia/clitoris, thinning of the genital skin, bleeding after intercourse, urinary/ bladder symptoms, urinary tract infections, incontinence and discharge.

I understand; it's not an easy topic to bring up and can be quite embarrassing. But addressing these concerns is crucial for getting the help you need. It's upsetting to think quite how many women suffer in silence!

The British Society for Sexual Medicine reports that up to 84 per cent of postmenopausal women have symptoms associated with GSM[9] yet only a minority receive any treatment.[10] Women who have received cancer treatment have an even higher risk. At every workshop I speak to women with all types of cancer who struggle very severely with these symptoms, and few have had any help.

GSM symptom checker

Symptom	Not at all	A little	A lot	Comments
Vaginal and vulval dryness				
Soreness/pain				
Irritation				
Burning				
Vulval skin tearing/splitting				
Labia and clitoral shrinkage				
Discharge				
No periods/ changes to period				
Bleeding after intercourse				
Painful intercourse				
Urinary tract infections, sometimes recurring				

Symptom	Not at all	A little	A lot	Comments
Urinary incontinence				
Urinary frequency				

Understanding where you are now to plan your next steps

Well done for taking time for yourself and going through your symptom checklist. How are you feeling now? If you have worked through your symptom checker and you're feeling a little overwhelmed, then this is totally normal. Really looking at our lives and what is going on can feel 'a bit much', especially as we have all come such a long way. Or it might feel good to get it all down on paper. This can be your first step towards putting together a plan for yourself. For now, try to remember that you don't need to know what to do about all your symptoms – we will take it one step at a time as you work through this book.

While you are doing this exercise, try to be as non-judgemental as possible. I have sat with hundreds of women working through this, and I've seen how self-judgement and unhelpful thoughts often creep into the conversation. By the time I meet with women, it is often a few months, or years even, after their active cancer treatment has finished, and a common thread is that people think they should be doing better than they are. They feel as though what they are experiencing isn't normal, that it's just them. But cancer treatment-induced menopause is a challenge in so many ways, and having many symptoms is a normal reaction to the physiological state your body has been put into. I'd argue that what's not normal is that you have had very little to no help so far.

There's a societal and personal expectation that, once active cancer treatment ends, we should 'move on' and feel 'back to normal'. It's common to believe that finishing treatment means everything should be better. But if no one in your medical team prepared you for the possible long-lasting effects of menopause – persistent and severe symptoms – it's completely understandable that you feel as though you should be 'doing better' than you are. Women tell me that no one prepared them for the effects of surgical menopause or that they were told to 'just take this little white pill (tamoxifen), which most people tolerate very well.' There is a huge gap between expectation and reality and it's really frustrating to see, as it can easily lead to self-blame and feelings of inadequacy. But please know you're not alone in this.

People often say, 'Cancer is the gift that keeps on giving' and I agree, especially when ongoing menopause symptoms make life difficult. Plus, there comes a time when, even though you're now dealing with menopause symptoms, you might not want to sound like you're complaining.

You and your mental and physical body have gone through a huge trauma and much change. From your body to your hormones all the way through to your soul, you've been affected and altered. For now, you've done wonderfully. You've taken the brave steps to look back, reflect, dream of how you want to feel and live, and evaluate your current experiences by filling in the menopause symptom checker. This process is absolutely crucial for becoming an empowered patient. By gaining a clear understanding of your journey so far and where you are at right now, you can arm yourself with the knowledge and confidence to advocate for your needs and make informed decisions to figure out your next steps towards feeling better. You really do deserve to feel supported and to get the help you need to manage your menopause after your cancer diagnosis. And it starts with you, here, today.

REFLECTIONS

1. Give yourself credit and a big pat on the back for everything you have been through and are doing.
2. Did you know about all the symptoms associated with menopause before? Or were you surprised at quite how many symptoms there are?

POSITIVE ACTIONS

1. Fill in your menopause symptom checker.
2. Once you've completed the checker, put a date in your diary to repeat the exercise in six weeks' time.
3. Treat yourself for taking action – maybe buy a new notebook or a special tea; that way, you'll have something enjoyable to look forward to the next time you sit down to track your symptoms.
4. Connect with others: consider reaching out to a friend or loved one, and sharing some of your experiences.

CHAPTER 3
HOW TO NAVIGATE THE MEDICAL SYSTEM

When I first began to prepare for how to manage my upcoming surgical menopause after breast cancer, I had no idea where to turn for help. I wasn't under the care of my oncologist or surgeon any more, and I felt lost trying to figure out which doctor could support me. Many people I speak to echo this experience: 'I have no idea where to turn for help.'

While this chapter is dedicated to helping you navigate the medical system – so you can identify the right experts, ask for the right support and understand what you might expect along the way – today, when I get asked about the best way to tackle menopause after cancer, I always advocate for a holistic and collaborative approach.

For me, a holistic approach means looking at your health and wellbeing from all angles, rather than relying on a single solution. Menopause after cancer is complex, and, in my opinion, there's no one-size-fits-all answer. A holistic approach involves considering your physical, emotional and mental health as interconnected parts of your recovery and wellbeing. The next chapter will explore this in more detail, including all the additional tools – besides medicine – in your menopause after cancer toolkit.

A Patient and Doctor Collaboration

Your doctors can offer guidance, essential treatments, medications and medical expertise, but there's also so much you can do on your own to improve how you're feeling. You'll most likely need a bit of both.

For this collaboration to work well, both sides need to recognise their roles. While your doctors offer their medical expertise and support, you bring your intimate knowledge of your body, your needs, your wishes and your life. And ultimately, you are in charge of 'project you', because you know yourself best. You know what you're experiencing, how much or how little your symptoms affect you, what's important to you, and you understand what worries you, as well as your hopes and wishes for the future. Your responsibility is to communicate these things clearly, and your doctors' responsibility is to listen and respond in ways that meet your needs. If this patient–doctor collaboration is mutually active and successful, it will mean you can make informed decisions together.

For me, truly understanding this active partnership did not happen until long after my initial diagnosis. The early days of cancer treatment, chemotherapy, radiotherapy and surgeries felt passive. I went from one appointment to another and I thought my doctors knew best. Wanting to be the good patient, I hardly asked any questions. It took years for me to fully grasp my agency and my potential to make a real difference to how I was feeling physically and mentally. I also learned how to navigate the medical system, and was determined to find out who could support me with what symptom. This became the 'active part' in my healing. No one ever tells you how to put together your medical team or how to live your life after cancer, and so I realised I had to become actively involved in my recovery and take charge of that part. I started to ask more questions of my doctors, and at the same time I chose to look after myself in ways that worked for me. I had to put together my own recovery and wellbeing strategies – and, of course, there was a lot of trial and error. And although I realised that I couldn't control everything, I discovered that I did have the power to influence my day-to-day wellbeing in positive ways. On some days this was by eating nourishing foods, or going to counselling; on other days it was by advocating for myself and asking for a second opinion. I believe that we have the power to influence how we are feeling on most days in different, even if just really small, ways.

Becoming 'active' in how to string together your care providers and how you support yourself will take time, and it might come more naturally to some than others. Many people I have worked with have had a little voice of doubt telling them they are not worthy of voicing their needs, they 'don't want to be a bother'. If you have a voice like that, I am here to tell you – you fully deserve your own love and care, as well as the care and support of others.

I am sure many of you reading this feel you are far from being in a collaborative relationship with your doctors. I understand. You might be thinking, 'I can't even get through to reception to book a doctor's appointment, let alone see a doctor face to face,' or, 'My next follow-up appointment isn't for months – what do I do in the meantime?' Many say, 'No one in my medical team seems to be able to help me with my menopause symptoms.' I hear you. The challenges in accessing care can be immense. Let's dive in.

Whose Job Is It to Help Us?

Do you know who in your medical team is equipped to help you manage your menopausal symptoms after a cancer diagnosis? If medical treatments have plunged you into menopause, surely someone in your medical team should take responsibility for assisting you, right? If your cancer treatment was years ago and you now need help with menopausal symptoms, shouldn't you be considered a complex patient who can access specialist care?

When did our medical system become so compartmentalised that it considers it normal to remove a woman's ovaries without helping her manage the sudden, severe onset of menopause? How can doctors prescribe endocrine medication for five to ten years with little to no explanation and then provide no access to support? Why would anyone think it's okay to tell women to come off their HRT immediately without offering any alternative options and guidance? You deserve good care that addresses the full spectrum of your health and wellbeing, so that you can live as good a life as possible after cancer.

Unfortunately, in most patient pathways this isn't the case – not in the UK, the US, Australia or in many of our other communities. Most people I speak to say they find themselves in a big void, feeling left to deal with their menopausal symptoms alone.

I vividly remember one evening during our first Navigating the Menopause programme with the UK cancer charity Trekstock: Jemima Reynolds, who was head of programmes, and I were in a webinar with over forty young adults, all in their twenties and thirties, who had experienced early menopause or menopause symptoms due to cancer treatment. We heard story after story of how no one in their medical teams had addressed the significant impact of their early, medically induced menopause. The most common sentence we heard was, 'No one said it was menopause.'

Georgie was 26 when she was diagnosed with stage four Hodgkin's lymphoma, which is a form of blood cancer. She had chemotherapy and went for months without a period, but concluded that it was the chemo causing that. Sadly, Georgie relapsed, and her next stage of treatment involved a gruelling stem cell transplant. 'I had to sign this paperwork to say that I understand that the stem cell transplant can make me infertile. But in all those conversations when they said, look, this treatment is likely to make you infertile, no one said to me, that's the menopause. It was probably a little ignorant of me because I didn't realise what else would come with it. I didn't realise they were saying that I would be in menopause. Knowing that I was going to be in the menopause would have been really helpful because I thought I was losing my marbles. I had very low moods, I was unbelievably anxious, I had panic attacks. I didn't realise these were symptoms of the menopause.'

Georgie sought the help of a therapist and it was only from speaking to them that she worked out she was in the menopause. Upon being questioned, her doctors confirmed this was indeed the case. 'And then it made sense: the joint pain, the terrible memory, the night sweats. I mean, I went back to my professor at the hospital, saying, 'I'm having night sweats again. Does this mean the cancer's back?'

At the time I spoke to Georgie, no one had told her that she had access to a menopause specialist on the National Health Service, and she had received no specialist advice as how to manage her symptoms or look after her long-term health. She, like many others, fell into the void of menopause care. As Jemima said at our webinar, 'The onus should not be on the patient.'

Since then, I have heard hundreds of similar stories. Patients had to figure out they were in menopause on their own, or they were bounced between their GP and oncologist without getting help. I know that sometimes we hold back, not wanting to take up too much of our doctor's time or feel like a burden, but we must address our concerns. We owe it to ourselves and every woman who comes after us. Our conversations are going to shape and inform the way our doctors manage menopause after cancer for future generations, so the more we openly talk about our struggles with menopause, the more doctors will realise this is a healthcare issue that needs to be addressed from the get-go. I am convinced that these conversations, alongside the movement we have created, will also fuel new research and scientific advancements. As doctors and researchers become more aware of the widespread impact of menopause after cancer, they will be more inclined to explore better treatment options, improved therapies and new medications. So let's speak up.

Right now, I also believe we can't expect someone diagnosed with cancer to navigate these life-changing challenges on their own, so doctors, medical boards and organisations have to do better. I can't change the current system, but I will try to help you make it work better for you.

A Worldwide Puzzle

I want to provide you with a guide to the practitioners who are part of a cancer survivor's medical team. Depending on your diagnosis and treatment you may be interacting with all of them or some of them, and I will explore what role they can each play in supporting you with your menopause.

I live in the UK, so my expertise lies in how to help fellow survivors get the best out of the system here. I recognise that accessing menopause care is very different in different parts of the world, but you can map out a care plan for yourself using the information on the following pages by applying it to the medical system wherever you are in the world (and on pages 53–54 I've offered some helpful advice from two wonderful colleagues of mine for our US and Australian readers).

Connect to Your Healthcare Team

Oncologist/surgeon

If you're under the care of an oncologist or surgeon and are starting treatment, make sure to ask these questions very clearly:

- Is this cancer treatment going to induce menopause?
- Please talk me through what symptoms I may experience.
- Where do I go for help if I experience symptoms of the menopause?

If you're partway through your treatment, it is really important that you share your concerns, symptoms and wishes with your oncologist or surgeon. There is no way they can help you if you are not clear in expressing what is going on. When I was going through chemotherapy, all of my fingertips started to become very painful and, although my doctors had warned me that my nails could become discoloured, I never communicated this with them when my nails did indeed begin to change colour and some even fell off. I just wanted my oncologist to think that 'I'm doing super well, that I have got this!' Please don't ask me why – it's not like anyone was going to give me a badge for suffering in silence! I hid my hands and never asked for help. We know there can sometimes be a bit of 'white coat syndrome' – a tendency to feel nervous or hesitant around doctors – but try to remember that they are there to support you, and honest communication is key to getting the best care.

It probably also feels as though there is never enough time during your appointments and that there are other and maybe more important treatment decisions that have to be made. Appointments with our oncology team are often laden with anxiety, and if we're not prepared it is so easy to walk away from them thinking, 'I should have asked...' Filling in the symptom checker on pages 30–32 will help you to be much clearer in talking about your symptoms with your doctor, which is not only going to save some time but will also help you feel a little more in control.

Is it even our oncologist or surgeon's job to help us manage the symptoms of menopause?

Maybe it is, maybe it isn't. You might say yes, given the close relationship between cancer treatments and the onset of menopause. Or you might feel that oncologists and surgeons are cancer specialists and they may not have the expertise or time needed to properly address menopausal symptoms. While I believe there are strong arguments on both sides, I also feel that oncologists and surgeons should be involved in the initial discussion of treatment-induced menopause, and should adequately prepare patients for what they may be experiencing, managing expectations and making appropriate referrals. Most people I speak to say they wish they had known what to expect. For patients on endocrine treatment for hormone-sensitive cancers, maintaining an open conversation with their oncologist is crucial. I have spoken to fantastic oncologists who help their patients with tweaking their medication, swapping treatments around and making referrals to help them manage their side effects better. And I also know of patients who have stopped their medication altogether without even telling their oncologists because they feared they would not be heard and supported – or, worse, that they would be judged.

If you feel your oncologist or surgeon is too preoccupied with other, more pressing treatment decisions, you can always ask them who in their team might be best equipped to help you manage your menopausal symptoms. Cancer nurses are often very well equipped to help you manage the complex aspects of menopause.

Anne, a lady in her fifties who joined our menopause programme, was diagnosed with breast cancer and after surgery and radiotherapy was prescribed aromatase inhibitors to reduce her risk of a cancer recurrence. However, she had never seen an oncologist, and was merely handed a booklet about aromatase inhibitors by a radiotherapist. She was told all the information she needed was in there. She had no consultation about the drug and what the benefits and risks of it were for her, and she was too worried to start the medication due to the horror stories she'd heard about its side effects. This lack of support left her unable to begin a crucial treatment. Oncologist Dr Claire Macaulay explains that this isn't an isolated scenario: 'We do know that somewhere between 20–25 per cent will never actually start the medicine they're given.' Encouraged by our group, Anne realised she deserved proper information and wasn't a bother. She persisted, asked the breast nurse if she could see an oncologist, and, armed with more information, began taking her medication.

Anne's story shows that sometimes we just need a little encouragement so that we can show up for ourselves and advocate to seek the right care. Anne did not have all the information she needed to make an informed decision and start her medication. It was wonderful to see that she became more confident in asking for support. But of course I meet many people who have felt that they've hit a brick wall and who could not find the support they needed from a specific doctor. If this is your experience, try not to give up, and think who else in your medical team may be a good person to talk to.

Specialist nurse

Your specialist care nurse, or clinical nurse specialist, is the person most likely to have many answers for you and, as part of your cancer team, may be very well equipped to help you. You also probably have the most contact with your cancer nurse in the months after your active cancer treatment, which is the time when many survivors start to have menopause-related concerns and questions.

A few months after launching The Menopause and Cancer Podcast, I had an email from a wonderful specialist breast care nurse called Andrea Ward. Andrea is the team leader for the breast care nurse team at York and Scarborough NHS Trust in the UK. She was so passionate that more support was necessary that she shared her valuable knowledge from over twenty years' experience with our listeners, saying: 'After the initial treatment, many cancer patients face an entirely new challenge – menopause induced by their treatment or medication. It's not just a side effect; it's a life-altering experience that can be easily overlooked. While oncologists and surgeons may see the main treatment as complete, the reality is that living with the ongoing effects of menopause is a massive, often overwhelming, part of the journey. Our job as breast care nurses is to ensure that this isn't minimised. We are here to engage deeply with patients, to help them navigate this new normal, and to support them in truly living beyond their diagnosis. This isn't a side note – it's central to their wellbeing, and we're committed to being there every step of the way. You're not a bother – reach out to us!'

General practitioner (GP)

If you have been discharged by your cancer team, your general practitioner (GP) is going to be your first point of contact. And even if you're still under a cancer team, if you don't already have a relationship with your GP it's a good idea to start building one. Many women I speak to say they have not seen their general practitioner in a long time as they have been under the care of the cancer team at the hospital. But going forward, your GP can support you with treatment and referrals. Ask your practice manager who at your clinic has a special interest in women's health and menopause. Be direct: 'I've been diagnosed with cancer. Now I need help in managing treatment-induced menopause.' If you're experiencing early menopause (before the age of 45),[11] tell them: 'I need help with cancer treatment-induced early menopause. I'm young, and I know this is complex. Can you please tell me who the best person at the practice is to help me with this?'

Dr Lindsey Thomas, an experienced GP and menopause specialist with whom I've co-hosted many workshops for our groups, has shared her expertise on the subject, explaining to me that: 'GPs can play a role as an advocate for their patients, especially when it comes to navigating the complex landscape of menopause care after cancer treatment. If you know hormone replacement therapy is not contraindicated, for example, then your GP should be well equipped to talk you through all of your options – hormonal and non-hormonal.' In the next chapters I'll be exploring what these options are.

Your GP will also be able to help you look after your future health. You might want to have your thyroid, cholesterol or vitamin levels checked, or have other blood tests, and so this collaboration between you and your GP is important now as well as in years to come. It is worth it for you to put a bit of time into finding someone you feel can support you.

Menopause specialist

In my view, in the majority of cases but not all, specialised care is necessary to address the specific menopausal needs and concerns of people who have undergone cancer treatment. I will explain to you how you can access specialist care; however, I feel I must warn you that this is where you may need patience, perseverance and determination.

The British Menopause Society (BMS) states that: a menopause specialist is a healthcare professional who has additional knowledge and skills, assessing and treating women with complex needs, such as multiple treatment failures, POI, complex medical problems, high-risk cancer genes or hormone-dependent cancer. They accept referrals of more complex patients and support colleagues to manage patients with higher risk factors or where there are multiple factors that affect decision-making.[12]

In the UK, you are entitled to be seen by a menopause specialist on the National Health Service. During my conversation with Dr Thomas (which we have made into a YouTube episode; and I have linked to it in your digital handbook), she mentioned that cancer survivors often face unique challenges, and many require a thorough conversation with a doctor about their specific needs and treatment options. 'The limited number of menopause specialists in the UK leads to long waiting lists for appointments. However, while waiting for an appointment, patients can contact the clinic to be put on a cancellation list, or your GP can request advice and guidance from the menopause specialists to explore interim care or treatment options in the meantime,' she explained.

The waiting times for NHS menopause specialist appointments are currently long, ranging from 9 to 18 months, and some have to qualify to even get on the list. While I know how frustrating this is, I want to help you use this waiting time proactively, through both my guidance and the expertise of the experts I share in this book. By the time you have worked through the book and done some of your own research, you will be much more informed and educated, ready to discuss exactly what you need help with and what you want to address.

Let's turn this waiting period into an opportunity to empower yourself and take control of your health journey. And remember, the menopause specialist's help will only be one part of your toolbox – one of many! I completely understand that waiting for an appointment can be really stressful. That's why, later in the book, I write about a variety of proven strategies that our community has found helpful for managing anxiety, sleepless nights and other effects you may experience during that waiting time and making them a little easier to manage.

How to Find a Menopause Specialist

In the UK, the BMS (British Menopause Society) website has a 'find a BMS registered specialist' search option. You enter your postcode, tick NHS or private, and a list of specialists will be provided. There's still a bit of work to be done on your part, so read the next few pages for my tips on finding a specialist that's right for you.

You can be referred outside of your area, even outside of your county if you are willing to travel or if telephone appointments are offered, so don't think you have to find a clinic within a certain distance of where you live or where you were treated. However, not all clinics are able to take outside-of-area referrals, and sometimes the arrangements can be quite complicated. Also note that not all menopause specialists work in so-called 'menopause clinics'. Some are called centres for reproductive health, or you may be seen in gynaecological units. Don't be too put off by long waiting times – use the knowledge acquired from this book to start putting together your action plan for yourself.

Among the many comments in our Facebook community where people share their struggles, we also get some positive ones, and I wanted to share this one with you.

> *'I just wanted to share a really positive experience of seeing a menopause doctor on the NHS, to give those of you struggling some hope and also to quote what the doctor said to me: 'You have been through so much already with all the treatment. You absolutely deserve to be supported and helped with these debilitating menopause symptoms and that is why it is so important that we have clinics like this to support women like you.' My oncologist referred me to the menopause clinic, which is held once a week at the breast clinic. I have really been struggling with severe menopausal insomnia, hot flushes, migraines and no libido. My GP had been very helpful, but symptoms were getting worse, impacting my ability to work and function. When I sat down with the doctor she already had all my history of breast cancer, treatment, referral from oncologist, so I didn't need to go through all that. She wanted to know what I was struggling with. Just being listened to, heard, offered*

informed choices, really made such a difference. I literally burst into tears with relief. After struggling so long, I finally feel hopeful about the future. It's just a shame we are not given this support as part of our treatment and that we are left struggling for so long. I was 45 when I was diagnosed.' **Emma**

Dr Corinne Menn, a board-certified OBGYN and Menopause Society Certified Practitioner based in the US, says, 'The best place to start: find a clinician who *really* knows menopause. Oncologists are experts at managing your cancer and it is important to partner with them in survivorship, but let's be real – they're not usually the go-to experts for menopause or sexual health after breast cancer. That's where menopause specialists come in. The Menopause Society, formerly known as the North American Menopause Society (NAMS), has a list of certified practitioners. Another great resource is the International Society for the Study of Women's Sexual Health, where many members are well versed in both sexual health and menopause management.' (Both resources are linked in your digital handbook.)

Dr Menn continues, 'Before booking, call and ask: "Do you work with women dealing with cancer and menopause? How much of your practice is dedicated to menopause management?" Make sure they are board-certified in their speciality. Don't limit yourself – look into telehealth (virtual appointment) options, too!'

When I asked Dr Menn if she could give us even more specific advice, she wasn't hesitant to add, 'Now, here's the deal: you're the CEO of your survivorship. Prepare for appointments like you're walking into a board meeting. Bring a concise summary of your cancer history, including your pathology report (bring all the relevant information from your diagnosis), and a list of your menopause symptoms, plus anything you've already tried. Before you step into that office, think about your top one or two priorities. Start small. When you tackle one or two issues successfully, you build momentum – and that leads to big improvements in your health and quality of life. And know what you are asking for, don't be afraid to be specific and clear. If you're stuck between conflicting recommendations, remind your docs about the principles of shared decision-making and informed consent. You're not asking for permission; you're seeking a partnership to make the best choices for *your* health.'

'In Australia, cancer patients are encouraged to seek support and referrals to a menopause specialist, such as a GP with expertise in menopause, an endocrinologist or a gynaecologist, through their multidisciplinary team (MDT). These referrals are most often provided by an oncologist, though an oncology nurse may also be able to offer advice and recommendations,' says Sonya Lovell, a breast cancer survivor, passionate advocate and our brilliant Menopause and Cancer ambassador for Australia, who is based in Sydney.

What can we learn from others' experiences?

At a menopause and cancer workshop I spoke to the lovely Kate, who was diagnosed with secondary hormone-positive breast cancer and was really struggling with many of the side effects of cancer treatment. Kate was telling me that, after attending a few of our online workshops, she had asked her GP to refer her to a menopause specialist. She was told that they only refer people who are on hormone replacement therapy and when it's not working for them – which is incorrect. Kate felt encouraged by what I had been sharing with the groups in our workshops, and made another appointment with a different GP, who was not reluctant at all and referred her without further discussion. This GP also reassured Kate that she herself had plenty of experience and in-depth menopause training to help Kate manage her menopausal side effects through some non-hormonal treatments.

I feel we can learn a lot from this example:

1. Persevere and advocate for yourself: don't be discouraged or brushed off. Whatever you feel you need to ask for, keep asking until you get the answers and support you deserve. It may take more than one go.
2. Find the right doctor: some general practitioners know more about knee injections, others know more about menopause. The right doctor can become a wonderful ally in your journey. I advised Kate to stick with her second GP, who seemed really well equipped to help her, and to request her for future appointments if possible.

The role of private medicine

Dr Lindsey Thomas thinks it is important to recognise the excellent care the NHS provides in the UK. However, due to the current demands on the system, there are often long waits to see a menopause specialist. If it is within your means, you may want to consider private medicine to avoid long waiting times for appointments. Private appointments offer more time and flexibility for longer discussions with specialists, which many women tell me is what they are seeking the most. 'I just want to be able to talk to someone who will listen and understands,' an attendee of a recent workshop said to me.

But not all private menopause specialists have adequate experience with cancer patients. When you choose a private menopause specialist, ensure that you email in advance, consider telling the practice manager a little about your medical history and ask them to confirm that the specialist you have chosen has adequate experience in working with people with cancer. Generally, a doctor who also works in a specialist NHS clinic may have more experience with complex cases, because NHS clinics often treat a high volume of complex patients, compared to those outside the NHS. Of course there are plenty of exceptions, so just make sure you do your homework.

Manage Your Expectations

Like anything, liaising with your healthcare team is a process, and you need to manage your expectations. It may take several 'gos' and appointments. You will have much to discuss, much to digest, things to try, decisions to make, and you can't expect to walk away feeling 'sorted' after one appointment. If you choose to see a new doctor, they also need some time to get to know you. In many cases making difficult treatment decisions will require more than one conversation. The clearer you can be about what you want out of the appointment, the better and more helpful for your doctor. Give yourself and your doctors time to come up with a plan for you together.

Collaboration and communication

Successful treatment decisions thrive on collaboration and communication between patients, GPs, menopause specialists and oncologists. That's when we can each do our bit and contribute to our healing and recovery. We should all come together and, ideally, each practitioner should play a crucial role in helping you achieve a quality of life that feels right. Your suffering should not be seen merely as a side effect of cancer treatment that you have to put up with. Together, through adequate preparation, perhaps adjustments in medication, exploring new treatment options and continuously assessing your situation, you can strive for the best possible outcome.

Even in less-than-ideal circumstances, much can be done. Yes, navigating the medical system for menopause care after cancer treatment is challenging, but, by seeking specialised help, advocating for yourself and having open and honest discussions with healthcare professionals, you at least give yourself the best chance of accessing the care and support you need.

Dr Menn encourages us, 'Survivorship, cancer and menopause, it is a long and winding road that starts the day you're diagnosed. There will be detours and roadblocks to quality, evidence-based care, but keep pushing. You've already done the hardest thing – fighting cancer. You can manage the collateral damage, improve your health span (not just your lifespan), and decide how to balance it all based on your values and priorities.'

It's important to note that besides your oncologist, specialist care nurse, surgeon and GP, you will most likely ask for the help of other practitioners too at one point or another. So many of the people I speak to find value in using complementary therapies alongside their oncologist's treatments to help in their healing journey. When choosing these practitioners, the same principle applies as discussed above. Make sure they have adequate experience in working with cancer patients. I discuss the risks and benefits of these therapies in Chapter 8.

REFLECTIONS

1. Have you had the medical help you need from your cancer team to help with your menopause symptoms?
2. Do you have a good relationship with your general practitioner, or is this a good time to try to find a GP with a good knowledge of women's health issues and the menopause?
3. Right now, do you feel you could benefit from specialist help?

POSITIVE ACTIONS

1. Review your medical team. Is there a gap? What can you do to fill it? Contact somebody for further support.
2. Remember to fill in the symptom checker in the meantime and while waiting for appointments. This way, you'll be better equipped to ask the right questions and advocate for yourself during your appointment. It's all about being prepared!
3. You're never a bother! You deserve the right help and heaps of support.

CHAPTER 4
YOUR MENOPAUSE AND CANCER TOOLKIT

We've discussed how a strong patient–doctor relationship can benefit you and who in your medical team might be able to help you manage your menopausal symptoms. Now it's important to build on this foundation. Through my own experience as a patient and working with hundreds of other survivors who also found themselves in a complex menopause situation, I believe that no one medication, treatment or strategy is likely going to be 'the thing' that will help you manage menopause after cancer.

You will most likely need to draw from different toolboxes, often trying out different strategies to see what works, maybe changing plans and trying something else. Every time I facilitate a workshop, I am blown away by the many different approaches people tell me work for them, and I really believe that we all need to take a holistic approach to looking after our bodies post cancer and managing the menopause. This is where we are going to look at all of your evidence-based treatment options to help you manage your menopause symptoms after cancer.

While hormone replacement therapy (HRT) would be the first line of treatment for menopausal symptoms for most people, including those with premature ovarian insufficiency (POI),[13] you may have been advised not to take it, for example, if you have a hormone receptor-positive cancer. If this is the case, it is especially important to understand that there are many other tools you can work with.[14] The illustration below gives you an overview of the various options available to you – medical and lifestyle options and complementary therapies. We will look at each of the treatment options in detail in the following chapters. It is really important to me that you know you have options in managing your menopause symptoms, and this toolkit is here to help you find out what these are.

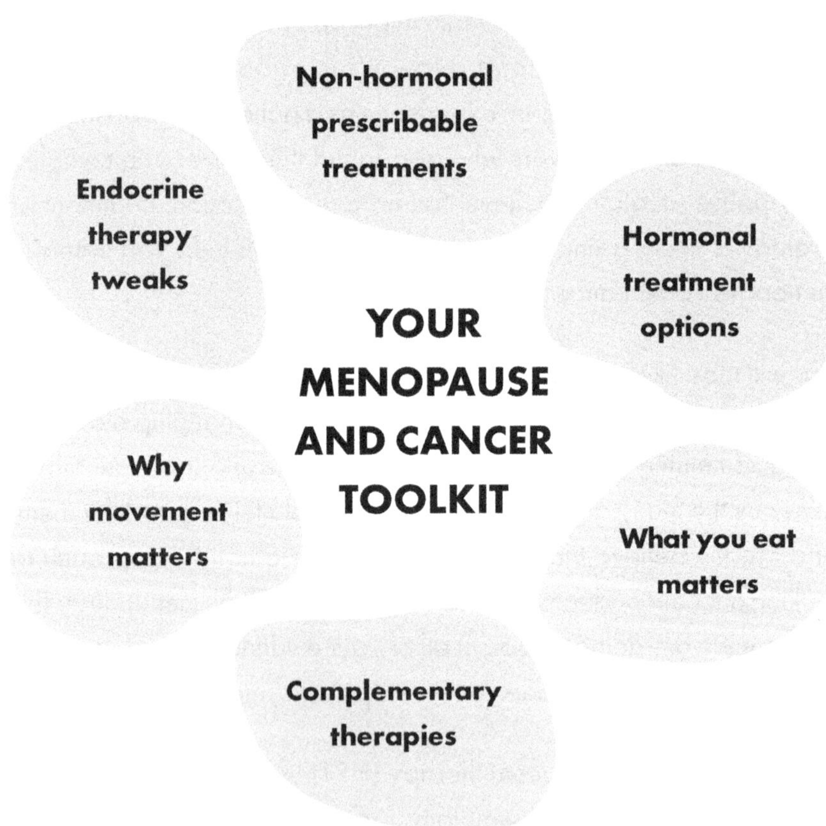

Holistic Healing

A holistic approach to healing is an all-encompassing approach that views you as a whole person, encompassing your physical, mental and spiritual health, rather than merely focusing on isolated symptoms or ailments or disease. Our mental health has an impact on our physical health and vice versa. Science tells us that stress can have such profound effects on our physical health. And I am sure you are well acquainted with the effect your physical health has on your mental health. It's huge, dealing with the anxiety, low mood, depression, fear and worry that can come as a result of becoming a cancer patient. Dr Annice Mukherjee writes in her book, *The Complete Guide to the Menopause*, 'Research has shown that chronic stress contributes to high blood pressure and furring of arteries, as well as raising the risk of heart attacks and strokes. It can also contribute to weight gain and the build-up of fat tissue in the body. It can even contribute to brittle bones.'[15]

Finding relief from menopausal symptoms will need to go hand in hand with healing and recovery from everything you have gone through, and often your life that came before cancer. Our bodies, minds and souls are so interconnected that we can't fully separate them. This means that healing and managing menopause after cancer will not simply be a case of finding the right medication or treatment. Your values, belief systems and how you're evolving as a person will play into and impact the treatment routes that resonate with you and what is right for you. I believe we need to pursue different options, weigh up our own risks versus our own benefits for each treatment and consider our personal preferences.

I, for example, feel very drawn to herbal medication and other complementary approaches, and that is probably for many reasons. I was raised in Austria, where pharmacies are full of herbal remedies, and doctors will often prescribe them for many ailments. I have seen first-hand how they work. Many of you reading this will have no connection to herbal medicine and will therefore find it harder to believe in its effectiveness.

Melissa joined our group on the empowered menopause programme. She was still going through chemotherapy when we met and the plan was for her to have monthly injections to switch her ovaries off after her chemotherapy ended. She told us that she really struggled with this idea as she was planning a post-cancer recovery life where she would go off and travel and live abroad for a while. This was really important to Melissa, so it opened up the idea of having her ovaries removed instead of switching them off with the injections. Her oncologist had little to say on the matter and just made a referral to a gynaecologist for her to discuss with them, so she's waiting for that. This is not stopping her though. She has spent time at sea completing the first part of her sailing training, and has arranged to be abroad for three months after that. Melissa did not know it at the time, but she was actively taking part in her recovery process and putting together her 'life after cancer' life. She started to plan how she wanted to live, and that is hugely empowering.

What I feel we can all learn from Melissa's story:

- Healing is more than just recovering from surgery – it is also about daring to live a life after diagnosis, the best way we can.

- How unique we all are and how our values and what we want out of life will impact our treatment decisions.

- It's so important to go after what is important to you.

The Right Tool for the Right Time

You are in an evolving landscape of managing life after a cancer diagnosis. Your symptoms will change and your approach to addressing them will also have to alter. You as a person will change, and over time your strategies for coping will have to change and adapt too. Embracing this evolution is critical. Keeping an open mindset will allow you to reassess how you are feeling and encourage you to re-evaluate your treatment options and draw upon new strategies that will serve you at any given moment. What works in spring might not work in autumn, and the decisions you make one year might need to be adjusted the next. Besides, what you want out of life will change too – the 'you' that makes decisions just after active cancer treatment is most likely going to be a different 'you' to the person a few years down the line. I remember quite a few years on from my diagnosis I went through a hugely intense period of anxiety. I was managing badly and it affected my appetite. I lost weight that I did not want to lose and it was affecting my everyday life. I had learned from the experts on my podcast that in some cases medication can be helpful. So, for the first time, nearly ten years on from my diagnosis, I asked my doctor to prescribe me something to help. You see, for years I thought that managing with techniques such as mindfulness, counselling and CBT was the right way for me. It took a lot for me to open myself up to other strategies. I realised that what worked for me before was not enough now. I re-evaluated my options. And I'm so glad I did. Today I no longer take the medication, but, should I find myself in a period of heightened anxiety again, I will think about what I might need at that moment in life. Always go back to the drawing board – this will serve you the best.

Helen, a lady who was a few years into taking tamoxifen after active treatment for her breast cancer, told me: 'I had acupuncture and it seemed to help my hot flushes, but I'm just so busy now and haven't been back in a long time.' Helen had found a strategy for helping manage her hot flushes but, as her symptoms improved and life got more busy, she became a little less compliant. This is my gentle reminder to you that, as with taking any other medication, for your treatment routes to work you need to be consistent with them. You wouldn't expect your thyroid medication to work if you'd not been taking it, and it's the same with yoga, acupuncture and diet. We have to be consistent: to take ourselves to appointments, to fork out time (and sometimes money) for us to reap the benefits of our investment of that time.

As much as I believe this is the case, I also understand that trying to adopt lots of strategies can feel far too much at times, and you may not have the energy to do anything at all right now. Remember, this book is here to present you with your options, but you need to work at your own pace and within your means.

Connect to Others in Our Community

I hosted a workshop with a group of breast cancer survivors who were facing various stages of cancer treatment and menopause. One participant was struggling with the side effects of tamoxifen and had never spoken to anyone with a similar experience. Another person, recently diagnosed and awaiting a mastectomy, was distressed about having to stop the HRT that had helped her so much. Other attendees were a couple of years into their journey; all were on endocrine treatment and had been advised that HRT was contraindicated for them. And almost all of them followed the social media accounts of doctors who advocate for HRT education, and celebrities and friends who say how transformative HRT has been for them. But this focus on HRT was redundant for them. One lady, suddenly, feeling encouraged by being in a group of people that was 'like her', said, 'It really frustrates me that all my friends say how amazing HRT is and I can't have it!' Almost all of the others echoed how she was feeling and were so grateful that someone had spoken up. And so we talked about that, and the group felt huge relief in knowing that they were not alone. Surround yourself with people who get you and your situation. What's the point in surrounding yourself with the stories of healthy perimenopausal and menopausal women? Yes, there is some shared experience, but you are a much more unusual case with really specific requirements. Tune in to the stories of other survivors and draw from their knowledge and strength. Our Menopause and Cancer chat hub on Facebook is a great place to start. I've linked it in the handbook.

Become Your Own Cheerleader

I hope you find plenty of inspiration in this book to spark your own menopause management action plan, filled with treatments and strategies that work for you. You may feel excited and motivated as you start this journey, and that's wonderful, but let me tell you, it's normal for motivation to dip along the way. When it does, pay close attention to how you speak to yourself.

It's easy to fall into a pattern of self-criticism during moments of overwhelm. Do thoughts like these sound familiar? 'I'm so lazy.' 'I knew I wouldn't stick with this.' Or, 'I always start something and then give up.'

If they do, know that you're not alone. These thoughts often sneak in when we're trying to make big life changes, especially after everything we've been through. But this is exactly when self-compassion matters most. Remember, you've already overcome so much. Be kind to yourself.

American podcaster Brené Brown wisely said: 'Talk to yourself like you would to someone you love.' Imagine encouraging a dear friend who's feeling overwhelmed. Would you berate them or lift them up? The same kindness should apply to you.

This journey isn't about being perfect; it's about making progress, one step at a time. Even small actions add up, and it's okay to pause, reassess, and start again when you need to. Positive self-talk and affirmations can be powerful tools to keep you on track. I've personally found that affirmations, which are simple, uplifting statements repeated regularly, helped me stay focused and motivated.

Most importantly, remember: you don't have to do it all at once.

Positive affirmations

A positive affirmation is a short, powerful statement that you say to yourself to encourage positive thinking and self-empowerment. It's something you want to happen, but it's written or said in the present tense – so as if it is already happening. If you are lacking in motivation, for example, then you would say, 'I am showing up for myself with all my energy and all my might,' or 'I am on the right track.' The statements are designed to challenge negative thoughts and beliefs, helping you to focus on your strengths and the good things in your life. If you are lacking in confidence for example, it can be as simple as writing 'I am confident.'

One of my favourite affirmations when I was recovering from surgery and treatment was, 'With every day, in every way, I am becoming healthier and stronger,' or simply 'I am healthy and strong.' If you are having to make tricky treatment decisions, you can say, 'I trust myself to make the right choices that lead to positive outcomes.' Telling yourself, 'I've got this,' can help you feel stronger and ready to take on challenges.

For me, repeating affirmations several times, over and over, also helped anchor me into the present moment, easing my anxiety. 'I am calm, centred and grounded' is one I repeated a lot. Perhaps pick one of the affirmations, or write your own and stick it on a Post-it note around your house or in your notebook, for example, to remind yourself.

Pick one of the below affirmations or write your own
• I am strong and resilient. • I honour my strength and healing. • I embrace positive change. • My mind is calm, my heart is open. • I attract positivity and radiate confidence.

REFLECTIONS

1. Take a moment to consider whether you are more drawn to certain tools. For instance, do you feel you would like to know more about medical treatments or complementary therapies right now? Or would you like to focus on your diet?
2. Which strategy have you tried so far to help manage your menopause symptoms? What has worked? What hasn't?

POSITIVE ACTIONS

1. Practise speaking to yourself as if you are your best friend. Say something kind or encouraging to yourself.
2. Choose or come up with a couple of positive affirmations and write them down somewhere you can see them.
3. Start with the chapter in this book that catches your interest most – whether it's how exercise can ease menopause symptoms or another strategy that speaks to you. Follow your intuition and dive right in!

CHAPTER 5
NON-HORMONAL PRESCRIBABLE TREATMENTS

Many people with a history of cancer are told that hormone replacement therapy (HRT) is not an option for them, and the conversation ends there. However, just because hormone replacement therapy may be contraindicated, this doesn't mean there aren't other medications that can help. If your doctor has said, 'I'm sorry, you can't have HRT,' and you are curious about what other prescribable options are out there for you, this chapter is for you. Even if you are currently on HRT, it's worth taking a closer look, as some of these medications can work well alongside it.

There is a variety of non-hormonal options available on prescription for managing menopause symptoms after cancer treatment; they can help target hot flushes, mood swings, anxiety, sleep, bladder and vaginal problems, and improve overall quality of life.[16] If HRT is not an option for you right now, your doctor can try to find a prescribable alternative that tackles hopefully more than one of your symptoms – which is why it is so important to fill in your menopause symptom checker. The clearer you can be about your symptoms and how they affect you, the better your doctor can then try to help you find a suitable prescribable medication.

As with any medication, there are risks and possible side effects and, of course, hopefully benefits. Most of the time, when I go through the prescribable list of non-hormonal treatment options at a workshop or webinar, I can see people furiously taking notes and then some will say, 'But I really don't want to use any more medication.' Of course, it's normal for people to feel this way after chemotherapy and all the other drugs that may have been put into their bodies. Or they'll say, 'I'm really worried about the side effects,' and, 'Will I feel worse before I feel better?' And that's totally normal too. Others say, 'I'll have it all, thank you very much.' There's nothing wrong with that either. That's where *you* come in again. What's important is that you know these options are available to you, that they can be helpful strategies and that you can explore them whenever the time is right for you.

Of course, you could simply look at some guidelines for prescribable alternatives to hormone replacement therapy, for example, and take that to your doctor to discuss. But I know that facts and figures alone are usually not enough to make decisions. People with – and without – a cancer diagnosis don't make decisions purely based on facts and evidence, because emotions such as fear, personal experience, bias and social influences often play a significant role in shaping our choices too, which is why I believe it's important that I also include some of the thought processes, worries, successes and failures from some of the brilliant people who have shared their stories with me. It's not lost on me that, for every example of a medication working well for someone, there's another example where it doesn't. I understand how frustrating and unhelpful this can feel when you're looking for solutions. This is why it's pointless to compare yourself to others – everyone's experience is different. You might fall into the majority or minority when it comes to experiencing side effects, but when something affects you it is always 100 per cent of your reality. Many people naturally seek reassurance, which I completely understand.

In this chapter, I share insights from Dr Alison Macbeth on what's available, along with her perspective on the pros and cons of these medications.

Non-hormonal Medication

Antidepressants

If you've been following the general menopause conversation, you've likely heard that antidepressants are not the first-line treatment for menopausal low mood or anxiety; HRT is. It's no surprise, then, that if you go to your doctor with a history of cancer after experiencing mood changes, anxiety, hot flushes, joint pains and other symptoms, and your doctor recommends an antidepressant, you might walk away feeling fobbed off or, even worse, think that you've been prescribed the wrong medication. Many people tell me, 'I know I'm not depressed, so why should I take an antidepressant?'

However, if you have had a hormone receptor-positive cancer and HRT is contraindicated, an antidepressant can be a valid treatment option. Some women even take antidepressants alongside HRT, and they do have their place in menopause management. While antidepressants are generally used to treat anxiety and depression, they can also be effective for certain menopausal symptoms. They are usually prescribed in lower doses, and different types can help with different symptoms. Getting them prescribed does not mean your doctor thinks you're clinically depressed; it means they are considering a broader range of options to help manage your symptoms. 'I always reassure women that we are not using high-dose depression quantities and we are giving them a much lower menopause dose as we are treating menopause symptoms and not depression,' adds Dr Macbeth.

The two most common types of antidepressant are: selective serotonin reuptake inhibitors (SSRIs) and serotonin-norepinephrine reuptake inhibitors (SNRIs).

Which type of antidepressant will be prescribed for you will depend on the symptoms you present with and also what other types of medication you are on. Remember not to skip the symptom checker exercise on pages 30–32. This is crucial to help your doctor decide what best to prescribe for you.

Different antidepressants have slightly different effectiveness and, as with most medications, what works for one person might not work for the next. Some antidepressants should not be used if you are taking tamoxifen; these include paroxetine, fluoxetine and high-dose sertraline and duloxetine.[17] Your doctor will know which ones are suitable for your health status and needs.

In general, antidepressants can improve quality of life, low mood, anxiety, hot flushes and sweats, and joint pains. However, it's crucial that you thoroughly understand from your doctor how they might benefit you and what the potential side effects could be before you embark on a course. It may take a while for antidepressants to work, and side effects such as nausea, dry mouth, dizziness, weight gain, headaches and anxiety are common in the first few weeks, until they tend to calm down. The general advice is to persevere for three months to determine if the medication is helpful. However, long-term side effects can include sexual dysfunction, problems reaching orgasm or a decreased sex drive, so if this is also a concern of yours, which it often is for women in our community, it is important to tell your doctor.

Communicate all your thoughts and worries to your doctor – from side effects to worries about being judged or even perceived as weak for needing help. There is much to consider. Everything is interconnected – a positive effect on one symptom might lead to a negative effect on another; therefore, it's essential to be clear about your current priorities.

Keeley emailed me saying how she felt left out of the wider menopause conversation and how glad she was that she had stumbled across my page on Instagram. Later, she joined our Empowered Menopause After Cancer programme, even joining me as a podcast guest, and it was wonderful to get to know her. She is an acupuncturist and a single mother, and had been suffering from severe physical and mental symptoms since her surgically induced menopause for ovarian cancer. Her doctor told her that HRT was not advisable and that there was no menopause clinic at the hospital, so she had no menopause help after her operation. Hot flushes were the worst symptom for Keeley. 'They were unlike anything I'd ever experienced. They were really volcanic. They came from really deep inside. I would sweat in between my fingers, the roots of my hair. They often came with a feeling of panic. I also had urinary tract infections, which were just awful and nothing I ever suffered from before. I was also struggling severely with anxiety; I felt fear and confusion. I felt foggy in my brain. I felt completely at sea. I even had a couple of panic attacks when I was driving. I was stuck in this really broken body. My joint and muscle pains had become crippling. I could barely walk.'

During one of our calls, we discussed antidepressants, and I explained how they could help with a variety of symptoms. Others shared their experiences too. At the time, Keeley was hesitant about taking more medication, worried about feeling worse before feeling better and concerned that the drug might make her feel 'like a different person' and 'not like herself'. She said, 'I just can't afford to feel any worse than I already do; I don't think antidepressants are for me.'

> *About nine months after the programme ended, Keeley called me. Her symptoms had worsened, and after yet another doctor's appointment she had decided to start a low-dose antidepressant. Despite her initial fears, Keeley told me the drug did the opposite of what she feared: it helped her feel much more like herself again, easing some of her debilitating symptoms. 'One of the first things that improved was my joint and muscle pains.'* **Keeley**

Keeley's example is not here to convince you how good antidepressants are. For every person who benefits, there is likely someone who doesn't. What her story demonstrates is that surgically induced menopause can be really tough and that, whatever your biggest worries are around trying different medications, they may not actually happen. We just have to try things to know what the benefit is for us. 'Although many women are frightened to use antidepressants, they are often worth a try. If you feel better and sleep better, then you may feel more able to make positive lifestyle choices such as exercise and healthy eating, which can in turn improve your joint pains, for example, and quality of life,' says Dr Macbeth. And sometimes it doesn't work out, but at least we've tried! Keeley's example also shows that it takes quite a bit of time until one actually makes a decision and then acts on it. And that's perfectly okay and normal. You are gathering information, digesting it and weighing up the pros and cons of a course of action. You might make up your mind, then change it again – you are embarking on a process. From the moment you start reading this book, to deciding on the best course of action for yourself, to finally making a doctor's appointment, quite some time may pass. It's important to remember that this is all part of the process. Taking care of yourself is a journey, and every step, no matter how small, brings you closer to figuring out what's right for you. Be patient and kind to yourself as you move forward.

Oxybutynin

This medication is normally prescribed to treat an overactive bladder, but it can also help to reduce the severity and frequency of hot and cold flushes. If, for example, your symptoms include hot flushes, night sweats and bladder symptoms, and you and your doctor are exploring non-hormonal prescribable options, then oxybutynin might be worth considering. Since this medication is being used for menopausal symptoms and not what it was initially designed for, doctors prescribe it as what's called 'off licence' for this purpose. Side effects may include stomach pain, diarrhoea, nausea, headaches, dry mouth and dry eyes.[18]

While discussing prescribable non-hormonal options at a workshop, a breast cancer survivor who was told HRT was not an option for her said she had been prescribed something for her hot flushes, but could not remember the name of the medication. Julia told us that she had not started taking the drug, despite having collected it from the pharmacy, and that it had been sitting in her bedside table drawer for the past few months. When I went through the list of prescribable options and mentioned oxybutynin, she exclaimed, 'That's the one!' She confirmed that bladder issues and hot flushes were her main symptoms, and also told us that she had tried antidepressants in the past – before cancer, even – and did not get on with them.

What we can learn from this example is that, with more time to discuss her medical history, her current symptoms and her doctor's advice, everything started to make sense for Julia. Given her poor experience with antidepressants, alongside her symptoms, it became clear why oxybutynin was a viable option and why Julia's doctor had prescribed it.

What was lacking for her was adequate information, and that was why her medication was sitting at home tucked away in her drawer.

Our doctors' appointments are so short, we're often nervous, and so it is common that we walk away feeling we've not quite had all the information we need.

When I look back at many of my own appointments I realise that, afterwards, I could hardly remember half of what had been said. I think an anxious mind can do that to you. For me, Julia's example really highlights how often we're just missing that final bit of information to help us decide what to do, leaving us feeling stuck and not taking any action. Since Julia's last doctor's appointment was several months ago, we agreed she would fill in a symptom checker and make another appointment with her doctor to understand more about the medication and its effects and benefits. She felt much happier with this plan and was reassured.

'I generally find that at the lowest dose most women tolerate this drug very well with few side effects apart from a dry mouth, which can be managed with a glass of water at the side of your bed. For a patient who cannot take HRT, for example, who presents with sweats, flushes and bladder symptoms, this medication would be my preference,' says Dr Macbeth. She adds, 'I do not, however, use this in older women (over 65) due to risk of falls and possibly reduced cognition.'

Gabapentin and pregabalin

Both gabapentin and pregabalin are medications classified as anti-epileptics. They are often used to treat other conditions, like nerve pain (neuropathic pain) and anxiety. You might wonder why these are listed here; but studies have shown that at certain doses they can also help reduce menopausal symptoms such as hot flushes. Gabapentin can also help with anxiety, joint pains and insomnia, which is often a big problem for those who are in treatment-induced menopause and for cancer survivors in general. Pregabalin can also lead to improvements in mood and wellbeing. Both medications come with possible side effects, such as a dry mouth, dizziness, drowsiness and weight gain. Additionally, both medications are considered to have a potential for dependence, which is why, in the UK, they have been reclassified as controlled substances due to the risk of addiction. The risk for dependency increases with prolonged use. As with all medications, it is important to follow the advice of the prescribing doctor when you want to reduce the dose or come off them altogether. Over the past few years, many menopause specialists have reported using these drugs less often than a low-dose antidepressant, for example, but they still have a place in some treatment plans.

Charlotte took to the chat forum and asked, 'I've just started taking gabapentin for the hot flushes. I was diagnosed with uterine cancer and was told I couldn't have HRT. I'm into week 2, so am up to my full prescribed dose. My question is, does anyone else taking it feel very emotional? I can be tearful at the slightest thing. My husband and I watched *Top Gun* last weekend and I was sobbing. Never have I cried at *Top Gun*! Is this because of the gabapentin thing or just a coincidence?' Other women in the forum agreed that they were also getting very emotional, and so Charlotte took the comments as an incentive to speak to her doctor again.

Charlotte's experience reminds me that it's very important to monitor your emotional wellbeing and symptoms when starting new medications. Sometimes we start to doubt ourselves and we wonder 'Is this normal?' By sharing her concerns and getting feedback from others, Charlotte made the decision to consult her doctor again. It does not matter if you think what you are experiencing is an unusual side effect or a common one. What matters is whether it affects you and bothers you. If it does, it should also bother your doctor. Sometimes we need to validate our own experiences by sharing them with others; this can really help and encourage us to take action and seek help. Trust your gut and trust yourself: you're not going mad; you're navigating something very complex and that can feel very confusing indeed.

'Although pregabalin is listed as an option on the BMS (British Menopause Society) website for the treatment of menopause symptoms, it is not recommended by the Menopause Society (USA) due to increased side effects. I therefore do not prescribe pregabalin. I prescribe gabapentin at usually low doses taken at night, as I find this helps my patients with sweats, insomnia and anxiety,' explains Dr Macbeth.

Clonidine

Clonidine is traditionally used to treat high blood pressure and attention deficit disorder. In the UK it is also licensed for the control of hot flushes and night sweats. It can cause side effects such as headaches and dizziness. These risks often outweigh the benefits, making it less ideal as a first-line treatment for hot flushes. But so many people have other health criteria that need to be considered – everyone is different, and what we very much need are options.[19]

For instance, someone recently shared, 'My doctor prescribed me clonidine for hot flushes. I'm very sensitive to medication – I can't take antidepressants and have tried oxybutynin, but it didn't suit me either. Has anyone had good results with this medication? I hate taking medication, but the hot flushes and lack of sleep are so debilitating right now that I'm almost at the point of trying HRT. Thanks for your input!' As you can imagine, we received a mixed bag of responses – some women found clonidine helpful, while others didn't experience the same benefit.

'The Menopause Society (USA) no longer recommends clonidine due to lack of evidence that it is effective enough given the side effects,' explains Dr Macbeth.

The key takeaway here is that what's most important is knowing that you have options.

Neurokinin 3 receptor antagonists (fezolinetant)

Fezolinetant is a new type of neurokinin 3 receptor (NK3R) antagonist used to treat moderate to severe menopausal hot flushes and night sweats. Fezolinetant is the generic name, and the brand name is Veozah. Many people call it a 'game changer', especially for those who cannot or choose not to take hormone replacement therapy. It was first approved in the US in May 2023 and is now licensed in the UK. At the time of writing, it is not yet available on the NHS but can be prescribed privately.

In spring 2022, just before the drug became available, I interviewed Professor Waljit Dhillo, a professor in endocrinology and metabolism, who had been involved in developing the drug at Imperial College London. Their research showed that oestrogen loss in menopause increases a hormone called neurokinin B. This hormone stimulates NK3 receptors in the brain's temperature-control centre. When oestrogen is low, this pathway becomes overstimulated. Blocking these receptors helps suppress the response and ease symptoms. Studies show NK3R antagonists can reduce menopausal hot flushes by 73 per cent, which is significant. So what about us cancer survivors?

I looked into what Veozah might mean for cancer patients. Some women I spoke to who tried it reported big improvements. But at present, there's no cancer-specific safety data, although studies are underway. Long-term data is also lacking, which makes some people uncertain.

Liver damage is a potential side effect, so liver function monitoring is recommended. In the US, insurance coverage can be tricky; in the UK, most people I spoke to accessed it through a private specialist and paid for the medication themselves.

Since that interview, I've had many conversations with women about this drug. Some are hopeful, while others are waiting for more research. Access and cost remain barriers in countries like Australia, Austria and the UK.

But now, some very promising news. A new study called OASIS 4 has provided the first data on a similar drug, elinzanetant, in women with breast cancer receiving endocrine therapy. The results are incredibly positive. Elinzanetant significantly reduced vasomotor symptoms in women taking tamoxifen or aromatase inhibitors. Benefits appeared early and were sustained over 52 weeks. It was well tolerated, with only minor side effects like headaches, drowsiness and diarrhoea.

Unlike Veozah, which targets NK3 only, elinzanetant blocks both NK1 and NK3 receptors. This may explain why it also helps with sleep. Encouragingly, no significant liver injury has been reported in the trial. While this drug is still in trial stages, it gives many of us hope that effective, non-hormonal options tailored for people during and after cancer treatment are finally on the horizon.

Non-hormonal Vaginal Treatments

Vaginal moisturisers and lubricants

Although we will cover vaginal treatments, with a special focus on vaginal oestrogen, in more detail in Chapter 6, it's worth noting that vaginal moisturisers and lubricants form an integral part of your non-hormonal vaginal treatments. Some can be prescribed by your doctor, which is why I wanted to include them here. As I said in the symptom checker chapter, despite over 80 per cent of women experiencing GSM (genito-urinary) symptoms, many find it difficult to discuss these issues with their doctors, resulting in them suffering in silence. Please address any of these symptoms with your doctor to get the help you need.

This is where vaginal moisturisers and lubricants come into play. It's something everyone can do to make a start on alleviating some of these awful symptoms. The most important thing about using products on the vagina or the vulva is that you have to be very careful about the ingredients!

In one of our sexual health workshops, sexual health educator Lavinia Winch, who is also a womb cancer survivor, said, 'Looking after our intimate health is important at all stages of our lives, from puberty through our reproductive and post-reproductive lives, whether we have had cancer or not. Knowing what's normal for us, and noticing any changes, allows us to seek help when we need it. We need to pay special attention to the health of our vaginas and vulvas because of the sensitive structure of the tissue and the susceptibility to infections such as UTIs, thrush and bacterial vaginosis (BV). No one should be washing their vagina – it is self-cleaning. However, if you want to wash your vulva, then it's important to use a product that is free of soap, glycerine and parabens and is pH balanced. Or simply wash with water or an emollient.'

Sam Evans, another brilliant sexual health educator and founder of adult toy business Jo Divine, with whom I have worked on several occasions over the years, says, 'Next, make it a habit to moisturise your vulva and vagina daily. For many cancer survivors, incorporating a vaginal moisturiser into your routine – just like you would with face cream – can make a big difference. Avoid any products that contain irritating ingredients. Stay away from glycerine, glycols and parabens, dyes, glitter and perfume. Frustratingly, even products prescribed by your GP may contain irritating ingredients, so look at the labels carefully.'

In the UK, a good skin-safe option your doctor can prescribe is the YES VM vaginal moisturiser and Hyalofemme.[20] In the US, Good Clean Love and AH!YES have great ranges of products. And of course, it's also about finding what works best for you! Doctors generally recommend using vaginal moisturisers as a long-term solution for managing symptoms of dryness and discomfort. Some may use moisturisers daily as part of their routine, while others might use them less frequently but consistently over time. Therefore, cost will be a consideration if you are paying for it.

Lubricants are not the same as moisturisers, although you'd be surprised how many people don't know there is a difference. Lavinia Winch explained this to us in a straightforward and helpful way. 'A vaginal moisturiser is for long-term, regular use to maintain moisture and comfort over time. On the other hand, a lubricant is for short-term use, typically before or during sex, to make it more comfortable by providing instant moisture. Using a suitable sexual lubricant can make a significant difference in comfort and pleasure during sex.'

Just as with moisturisers, ensure that the lubricant you choose is free from the harmful ingredients listed above. 'Become an ingredients detective!' Sam often says.

In the UK, you can get YES WB water-based lubricant on prescription. This is ideal for sex because it is pH-balanced and condom-safe, and has a light, natural feel. Sutil Luxe and Sylk are also good products, although not currently available on prescription. However, water-based products are absorbed quickly, so they may need reapplication. For those looking for something longer-lasting, oil-based lubricants, such as YES Oil-Based, provide protection against friction and discomfort as they soften into an oil and last longer. However, oil-based lubricants cannot be used with condoms, as oils can break down latex.

Everyone on the workshop was so grateful at the helpful advice and practical tips from Lavinia – and you can just imagine that we had quite a few giggles when Lavinia was discussing the 'double glide' technique. 'This involves applying an oil-based lubricant first for tissue protection, followed by a water-based lubricant to provide a longer-lasting, natural feeling. This combination is particularly recommended by gynaecologists and psychosexual therapists for those who experience discomfort during sex,' Lavinia explained.

The key takeaway is that moisturisers provide ongoing hydration, while lubricants offer immediate comfort for sexual activity, with the decision of whether to use water-based or oil-based options depending on condom use and the need for longevity. It's such important stuff – and honestly, none of it was on my radar before menopause decided to muddle into my life and stir things up.

If you try a regular routine of vaginal moisturisers for 6–8 weeks and do not find it helpful, you may benefit from adding vaginal oestrogen. This can be used alongside moisturisers and lubricants – more on that on pages 124–134.

Vaginal lasers

In addition to non-hormonal vaginal treatments such as moisturisers and lubricants, laser therapy has emerged as a promising option for managing symptoms of vaginal atrophy and dryness. However, it comes at a cost and is not available for most.

Laser therapy uses focused light energy to stimulate the vaginal tissues, promoting collagen production and improving the overall health and function of the vaginal walls. These treatments are often referred to as 'vaginal rejuvenation' and are performed by a healthcare professional in a clinical setting. Many women experience lasting relief from symptoms with periodic maintenance treatments. I have spoken to some doctors who are supportive of lasers for vaginal symptoms, others who are less so.

At the time of writing, laser treatments for vaginal health, such as MonaLisa Touch, FemTouch and Votiva, are generally not available on the NHS in the UK as the National Institute for Health and Care Excellence (NICE) has not fully approved vaginal laser treatments for routine use. NICE acknowledges that, while some studies suggest potential benefits, there is a need for more robust evidence to confirm their effectiveness and safety in the long term.[21] These treatments are considered elective and are typically provided by private clinics. Make sure you research a good provider who can give you the best care.

It may be helpful to bring these medication guidelines to your doctor to discuss your options. I've included the position statement of the Menopause Society in the US on non-hormonal therapy options,[22] as well as the BMS (British Menopause Society) document on prescribable alternatives to HRT,[23] in your digital handbook. These resources can help guide your conversation and ensure that you have the information you need to make an informed decision.

REFLECTIONS

1. There are a variety of non-hormonal prescribable options available for you to be considered should you wish to. From reading this chapter, is there anything you would want to explore further?
2. How would you feel about taking any medication? What are your concerns? What are the possible benefits?
3. It takes time to come up with a plan and you might have a series of doctor's appointments until you make up your mind. Do you want to get the ball rolling now and to make a doctor's appointment to discuss which treatments might be right for your specific needs?

POSITIVE ACTIONS

1. Continue to or start tracking your symptoms. Your symptom checker is on pages 34–35. This will help you in making more informed choices and communicating effectively with healthcare providers.
2. Schedule some research time for your healthcare so it doesn't feel overwhelming or take over your day. Instead of worrying about what you 'should be doing all the time, set aside 30 minutes later in the week to focus on it. Until then, give yourself permission to 'park those thoughts' and enjoy the present!
3. Download your digital handbook now, if you haven't already, to access the position statements and guidelines.

CHAPTER 6
HORMONAL TREATMENT OPTIONS

Given the debilitating menopausal symptoms many of the women I have spoken to experience after their cancer treatment, it is no surprise they wonder if hormone replacement therapy (HRT) could help them. But when it comes to women with a history of cancer, the question of whether to opt for hormonal options to treat menopausal symptoms and to help prevent long-term health risks such as osteoporosis – or not – becomes more complex. It is a nuanced decision, with competing factors to consider and weigh up. And of course, I know that many of you reading this have been told that HRT is not an option for you. Or you might not have a clue if it is or isn't. We need to understand our *individual* risks and benefits when it comes to taking HRT, while also considering our personal preferences. Most importantly, we deserve the answers that will allow us to make an informed decision about our health.

In this chapter I am going to start by explaining why the history of hormonal treatments is so mired in controversy for women across the world in general, as this will help us understand why we are on the back foot when it comes to discussing hormone replacement therapy for cancer survivors. I will also explore the various hormonal options available, from systemic hormones to local hormones. If you've been told you can't have anything with oestrogen, don't skip this chapter – especially the part on vaginal oestrogen. The conversation is much more nuanced than you might think, and there may be safe and effective options for you! And I'll delve into the scientific evidence – and lack of evidence – for hormone therapy after different types of cancer, in particular the use of HRT after breast cancer, which is a controversial topic. I hope the information in this chapter will form a starting point for a conversation between you and your doctor.

Experts, oncologists and menopause specialists whom I have spoken to have helped me compile the information in this chapter, in particular Mr Vikram Talaulikar. As an associate specialist at the Reproductive Medicine Unit at University College London Hospitals NHS Foundation Trust and an associate professor at University College London, Mr Talaulikar brings a wealth of expertise to this topic. He runs a busy NHS clinic where he and his team see many complex cancer patients. He is also one of our medical advisors at Menopause and Cancer, helping us to provide our community with accurate, up-to-date and evidence-based information.

What Exactly Do We Mean by Hormone Replacement Therapy?

Before we dive in, it's important to clarify exactly what we are referring to when we talk about hormone replacement therapy, because it can be a confusing world to navigate.

In the UK, we use the term hormone replacement therapy (HRT) when we talk about hormone therapy to treat menopausal symptoms. In the US and other countries, the terms menopause hormone therapy (MHT) or hormone therapy (HT) are most commonly used.

Hormone replacement therapy can be either **systemic** or **local**, depending on how the hormones are delivered and their intended effect. Systemic hormone therapy and local hormones are two very different things, and it's important that you are clear about each one's role in the body so that you can get the help you need. Just because you've been told that you can't have HRT may not mean you will not be able to use local oestrogen, for example.

Systemic hormone replacement therapy (HRT) is the administration of hormones, typically oestrogen, progesterone and testosterone, which are absorbed into the bloodstream and circulate throughout the body.[24] This type of HRT is the first-line treatment for menopausal symptoms and also for premature ovarian insufficiency (POI) and early menopause because it replaces the hormones that would normally be made in the ovaries. HRT is used to treat or alleviate a myriad of symptoms, including hot flushes, night sweats, vaginal dryness, mood swings, joint ache and many of the other symptoms we listed in the symptom checker in Chapter 2, as well as to prevent osteoporosis and heart disease associated with the lack of oestrogen.

Localised hormone replacement therapy involves the targeted delivery of hormones to a specific area of the body, typically the vagina or vulva, and there is minimal absorption into the bloodstream. This localised treatment addresses the genito-urinary syndrome of menopause (GSM), which I listed in Chapter 2. These include vaginal dryness, irritation, itchiness, painful intercourse, bleeding after intercourse, bladder symptoms and urinary tract infections.

HRT and its turbulent history

For some women, talking about HRT can throw up many different emotions. Some cancer survivors say to me that they are fed up of everyone saying how good they feel on HRT when they can't have it. Others tell me they were never contraindicated for HRT but, because no one in their medical team addressed their hormonal health with them, it took a lot of self-advocacy and time to have it prescribed. Some people feel that the potential benefits of being on HRT outweigh the risks for them, and they choose to take it even if it there is not good enough evidence for its safety. Many say they had no idea that local oestrogen was safe for them.

But most women simply say it's a really confusing topic and they have no idea where to begin to gather accurate information. As you'll learn in this chapter, much of the dilemma and controversy are rooted in a lack of robust and outdated data, and the fact that HRT has had a turbulent history in women's healthcare. My aim is to provide an informative, non-judgemental and objective overview of this complex issue, but, most importantly, to arm you with the information you need to start to understand whether hormonal treatment options may be right for helping you to treat your menopausal symptoms. Although you shouldn't have to, you may then need to advocate for yourself to gain access to it.

Hormone replacement therapy has had a rocky trajectory. It was first approved for use in the USA in 1942. In the 1980s its use rocketed when it was hailed as a revolutionary treatment for alleviating menopausal symptoms. However, in 2002, the Women's Health Initiative, a large-scale study in the USA funded by the National Institutes of Health (NIH), released results that dramatically shifted the perception of HRT. The study found that the combination of oestrogen and progestin (a synthetic form of progesterone) that was used in HRT, increased the risks of breast cancer, heart disease, stroke and blood clots in postmenopausal women. The media went into a frenzy. Almost overnight the narrative switched and women everywhere were told to stop taking HRT. The fear and confusion were overwhelming, and women were left to struggle with menopause symptoms on their own.

In the following years, investigators of the study published a further analysis of the trial, which revealed that the truth about HRT is much more nuanced and that some of the risks had been very much overestimated.[25] But by then the damage had been done and media reports trying to rectify the story never quite got the attention they should have done. Even now, many women are still reluctant to consider HRT despite experiencing menopausal symptoms, and doctors are often hesitant to bring it up. What makes this situation even worse is that the majority of doctors practising today have had little to no menopause training – something that astounds me. The truth is, the medical community and the media have let us down, and so many women worldwide have been left without the support they need. Only in recent years has HRT prescribing increased again, as the knowledge of and confidence in its benefits and safety have expanded to women across the world.

Why am I sharing this? Because when you consider that, from around 2002 until just a few years ago, HRT was rarely discussed as an option for managing menopause symptoms, and in fact menopause itself was not addressed either, it becomes clear why the conversation has been so limited – for all women, including cancer survivors. This often means HRT is simply dismissed outright rather than even being considered as an option. It is now up to us to become the campaigners of menopause care for cancer survivors. The confusion of the past, coupled with a lack of robust data, which I will go on to explain in detail, means cancer survivors are left to navigate menopause in a void. We are the generation in transit, waking up to the wrong reporting of the past, trying to undo what has been hard-wired into our generation and find the answers we need. Women's health has been overlooked and underfunded, resulting in gaps in research, awareness and access to comprehensive care. It is up to us now to get our voices heard so that our stories shape menopause care for cancer survivors in the future.

Addressing the Gap: Hormonal Care with a History of Cancer

During my time of working with people with a history of cancer who are also going through the menopause, I have come across so many who were not given the right help. I have met young women in their twenties who were left to suffer with post-cancer menopause symptoms and a detrimental effect on their long-term health despite having a medical history where systemic HRT was not deemed unsuitable.

There are simply countless heartbreaking stories of women falling through the gaps. Many of the women I speak to have done their research and were able to advocate for themselves. Yet, there are thousands who have no idea where to turn for information and advice. Not everyone can – or should have to – advocate for themselves. At so many workshops we've met women who believed they couldn't use any hormones at all, who had no one providing them with education on the safe use of localised vaginal oestrogen therapy, leaving some to suffer debilitating and dangerous recurring urinary tract infections. Local vaginal oestrogen, in many cases, is very safe and can alleviate these debilitating symptoms. Unfortunately, without this knowledge many women are left suffering, thinking they have no options.

We have also heard from oncologists who, only after suffering cancer-treatment-induced menopause themselves, started to change their practice to ensure their patients were adequately consulted on their hormonal health post-cancer treatment. Dr Rachel Elliott, consultant haem-oncologist at the Aneurin Bevan Health Board, told me: 'I'm a hospital consultant and look after cancer patients. I have no training in gynaecology and no training in menopausal management. My female patients would bring up their menopausal symptoms after their chemotherapy or after stem cell transplants, and very often I found myself saying, "Ask your GP for advice, it's not something I can help with." And now I'm going through treatment-induced symptoms myself, after my own cancer diagnosis, I can see how important it would be to be able to access help in one place and for oncologists or surgeons not to have to send people to their GP to manage their menopausal symptoms when we know they are most likely going to happen!'

> **'I had blood cancer and my chemo treatment put me into early menopause. No one in my medical team mentioned it was the menopause and, when I figured it out by myself, I asked my GP, who referred me to a gynaecologist. It's taken over two years and many doctors' visits to get the treatment I need.'**
>
> **Emily**

Dr Elliott's insights mirror what patients have been telling me. Women feel that they have had such good care from their cancer teams in helping them treat the cancer, but they feel they have nowhere to go for help with their, in some cases, highly distressing menopausal symptoms.

HRT Explained

I asked Mr Vikram Talaulikar, associate specialist at the Reproductive Medicine Unit at University College London Hospitals NHS Foundation Trust, to walk us through everything you need to know about hormone replacement therapy. He explains what it is, the different types and how to take it. On pages 104–108, he also provides a table to help you determine whether hormone replacement therapy may be appropriate after your type of cancer or when it's important to consult a specialist for further discussion.

Mr Talaulikar says,

> *'As outlined by Dani at the start of the chapter, HRT stands for hormone replacement therapy and here, I will explain to you everything you need to know about it. HRT replaces hormones that naturally decline during and after menopause – or, as in many cancer survivors' cases, rapidly decline because of cancer treatment. HRT typically includes oestrogen, progesterone and testosterone hormones (used alone or, often, in combination).*
>
> *It remains the most effective medical pharmaceutical treatment for menopausal symptoms and, if it is initiated before the age of 60 or within 10 years of menopause, it has several benefits, such as the improvement of menopausal symptoms, which leads to improved quality of life, bone mineral density preservation and protection of cardiovascular and metabolic health.*[26]
>
> *These benefits do, however, need to be balanced against common possible side effects, such as irregular bleeding, nausea, headaches, breast tenderness and long-term risks of thrombosis (blood clotting), breast cancer, womb cancer and recurrence of any previously diagnosed forms of cancer. Which hormones are used will be advised by your healthcare professional, taking on board your symptoms, preferences and medical history.'*

Which hormones make up HRT?

Oestrogen

Oestrogen is primarily produced in the ovaries, but some is also produced in our adrenal glands and fat tissue. It plays a crucial role in female sexual development and reproductive function – it regulates the menstrual cycle; but it also has many other vital roles: it maintains bone density; influences skin health and collagen production; affects mood, libido and cognitive function; and plays a role in cardiovascular health. Oestrogen interacts with different parts of the body by attaching to specific proteins called oestrogen receptors. We have these receptors all over the body, which is why a lack of oestrogen can cause such a wide range of symptoms. There are two main types of oestrogen receptor, and they can each have different effects depending on where they are, for example, in breast tissue, one type tends to encourage cell growth, while the other may help slow it down.

An understanding of how the receptors work will often help cancer patients make sense of their treatment, so, for example, some breast cancers are **hormone receptor-positive,** which means that their growth is influenced by hormones, such as oestrogen. These cancers have oestrogen receptors on their cells, and when oestrogen binds to these receptors it can promote the growth of cancer cells.

Oestrogen is a group of hormones that are primarily produced in the ovaries, but also in smaller amounts by other tissues in the body. There are four types of naturally occurring oestrogens: oestrone E1, oestradiol E2, oestriol E3 and oestetrol E4; each type is more prevalent at different stages of a woman's life and has specific roles.

HRT generally uses oestradiol processed from yams. It can be delivered via patches, gels, sprays, oral tablets or an implant.

If you still have a womb, oestrogen must be combined with some form of progesterone to protect its lining. This combination therapy is known as combined HRT. If you have had a hysterectomy, even if you have kept your ovaries, you can have oestrogen-only HRT. There are some exceptions, such as a history of endometriosis, or following a subtotal hysterectomy, where some of the lining of the womb canal may be left behind.

Body-identical vs bio-identical HRT: What's the difference?

It is important that we distinguish between the two types of HRT, as there has been some confusion about 'body-identical' versus 'bio-identical' HRT. In the UK, these two phrases refer to the following:

Body-identical HRT refers to licensed HRT that uses hormones that are chemically identical to those naturally produced by the human body. 'Licensed' means that the products have been approved by the Medicines and Healthcare products Regulatory Agency (MHRA) and are available on the NHS. It is this regulated body-identical HRT (rBHRT) that is commonly prescribed and which is what we are referring to throughout this book. Body-identical HRT includes various forms of oestrogen given through the skin, oral or vaginal route, and micronised progesterone.

Bio-identical HRT, on the other hand, refers to compounded HRT preparations that are not licensed by the MHRA. These are currently not recommended in the UK by the British Menopause Society as robust long-term safety data is lacking for many of them.

Progesterone

Progesterone is also produced in the ovaries, particularly after ovulation, during the second half of the menstrual cycle. Progesterone is crucial for regulating the menstrual cycle and preparing the uterus lining for pregnancy, and working with oestrogen to promote bone health. It also has a calming effect on the brain, which for some women can help improve sleep quality, regulate mood swings and reduce feelings of anxiety.

Its main role in HRT is to prevent oestrogen from overstimulating the womb lining and making it too thick, which can lead to endometrial (womb) hyperplasia or cancer.

Body-identical progesterone is available. Progestogens include both natural progesterone and synthetic progestins, which mimic its effects. Used in HRT and contraceptives, progestins act on progesterone receptors but differ in structure and may cause different side effects.

Body-identical or body-similar versions of progestogens include micronised natural progesterone and dydrogesterone; these appear to be safer than synthetic versions and have a lower risk of blood clotting or breast cancer with long-term use.

Other types of progestogens include norethisterone, levonorgestrel and norgestrel.

It can be delivered via tablets, patches, vaginal pessaries and the hormone-containing coil. The coil, also known as the Mirena or the LNG intrauterine system, can be used as the progesterone arm of HRT to protect the lining of the womb. The coil lasts five years for HRT and also provides contraception.

About 10–20 per cent of individuals suffer from progesterone sensitivity, which can make taking combined HRT challenging. Progesterone intolerance symptoms include headaches, nausea, bloating, breast pain, low mood, depressive thoughts, constipation, fluid retention and irregular bleeding. There are several options to minimise the impact of the progesterone part of HRT, such as trying different forms or routes of progestogens.

Testosterone

Testosterone is often thought of as a 'male hormone', but it is also an important female hormone, produced in the ovaries and adrenal glands. It helps regulate sexual desire, supports muscle mass and helps maintain strong bones. According to the UK's NICE guidelines, testosterone replacement can be offered to women with low libido when HRT alone isn't enough. Some also notice improved energy levels, better mood and less brain fog on testosterone therapy. However, more research is needed to confirm these benefits.

Testosterone is generally delivered through the skin. It is available as gels, cream and an implant.

It is used in small doses and does not usually cause side effects. Excessive use can cause oily skin, excess body hair, scalp hair loss and deepening of voice.

Testosterone can be added to any form of HRT, continuous combined or sequential combined (see opposite and page 100).

In the UK, testosterone is currently prescribed for women off licence, which means that it is used for a different purpose than that for which it was intended, as there is no product specifically licensed for women's use. Doctors often prescribe a low dose of a testosterone product intended for men, adjusting the dosage to meet the needs of women.

How do I take HRT?

I want to give you an overview of the most common ways to take systemic HRT if you and your doctor decide it's a good option for you. There are various formulations and dosages, and what you are prescribed will depend on your individual circumstances. It may take some time to find the right product and dosage for you, and in many cases you may need a few appointments with your doctor to find what works best.

- *Sequential combined HRT* is used for individuals who are in perimenopause and still have periods. You might have had cancer treatment that put you into temporary menopause, and then your periods came back. After that, you can go through perimenopause again, and may need help in managing your symptoms. In sequential HRT, you take oestrogen only for the first 14–16 days and then both hormones (oestrogen and progesterone) for the second 12–14 days. This usually results in monthly withdrawal bleeds, as the hormone regimen is designed to replicate the natural cycle and trigger a period. You can take testosterone additionally if you need it.

- *Continuous combined HRT* is more suitable for individuals who have not had periods for more than one year, or after the onset of menopause due to treatment such as surgery, for example. In continuous combined HRT, oestrogen and progesterone (and in some cases testosterone) are taken together daily and continuously. This means that there will be no monthly withdrawal bleeds.

Combined HRT (sequential and continuous) is associated with a slightly increased risk of breast cancer (overall extra risk of about 5–10/1,000 over 5 years).

- *Tibolone is another form of continuous combined HRT.* It is not a hormone on its own but has similar effects to oestrogen, progesterone and testosterone as it binds to their receptors in the body

- *Oestrogen-only HRT* is given to individuals without a uterus who do not need the progesterone part of the HRT. Oestrogen-only HRT is associated with no/minimal long-term risk of breast cancer.

When to start HRT after cancer treatment and why perseverance is key

When you start HRT will vary depending on your age, the type of cancer, treatment regimes used, background medical complexities and the nature of your symptoms. There are often good reasons why a particular formulation might be advised over another, and sometimes a formulation is prescribed only to be changed later if it does not suit you. Remember, finding the right approach can take time. Don't be discouraged – it's all part of the process of finding the most effective treatment for your needs.

HRT experiences: A brief overview

- The effectiveness and side effects of HRT can differ greatly from person to person.
- Some women are prescribed higher doses of oestrogen based on their absorption levels and response to HRT preparations, especially those who are younger.
- While some may absorb oestrogen from patches better, others may not find them useful and only absorb enough from oral or gel preparations of oestrogen, or vice versa.
- Oral tablets may not work for some, while implants may be the only form that work for others. This may be because of differences in hormone receptor distribution and drug metabolism between individuals.
- It may sometimes take a while, and trying two to three different HRT types, until a suitable combination is found. Don't give up!
- HRT is not a catch-all solution – it may be able to address many of your symptoms, but you may still suffer from a few.

Understanding HRT Options Based on Your Cancer Type

You might be asking if systemic HRT is okay for you after your particular type of cancer. And you may be curious about local vaginal oestrogen. The table on pages 104–108, compiled by Mr Talaulikar, gives an overview of which types of cancer get the 'green light' and can use systemic HRT post-diagnosis, as well as where systemic HRT is contraindicated. There is an additional column on the use of local vaginal oestrogen after each type of cancer, so that you have everything in one place. Also referenced are some types of cancers where robust data is currently lacking; and we delve into more details of HRT after breast cancer. For more detailed information about vaginal oestrogen, how it can help and the different types, turn to pages 124–134. I know this is a lot to digest, but we hope this information will help you and your doctors start a conversation.

Recommendations for the use of hormone replacement therapy by cancer type

The recommendations in the table overleaf are based on scientific evidence at the end of 2024[27] and may change as more research data becomes available in future. Recommendations are for general guidance only and may not apply to your individual case and unique clinical circumstances. Information relating to gynaecological cancers is based on the BMS (British Menopause Society) and British Gynaecological Society's guidelines for the management of menopausal symptoms after these types of cancer.[28]

Yes: Benefits outweigh risks

Discuss and individualise benefits/risks: Consider specialist advice to discuss

Avoid: Not recommended and refer to specialist advice

Type of cancer	**Subtype/ risk group**	**HRT recommendation**	**Vaginal oestrogen**
Brain cancer	Pituitary adenomas – including prolactinomas	Yes	Yes
	Meningiomas	Avoid	Yes
	Gliomas	Avoid	Yes
Malignant melanoma	Early-stage	Yes	Yes
	Advanced metastatic disease	Avoid	Yes
Thyroid cancer		Yes	Yes
Lung cancer		Discuss and individualise benefits/risks with specialist – can be used following some types but should be avoided after tumours that may respond to hormones	Yes
Stomach cancer		Avoid for oestrogen-sensitive tumours	Yes

Type of cancer	Subtype/ risk group	HRT recommendation	Vaginal oestrogen
Breast cancer	Hormone sensitive	Avoid	Yes
	Hormone sensitive – currently on tamoxifen	Avoid	Yes
	Hormone sensitive – currently on aromatase inhibitors	Avoid	Discuss and individualise benefits/risks with specialist
	Triple-negative	Discuss and individualise benefits/risks with specialist	Yes
Liver cancer		Yes	Yes
Pancreatic cancer		Yes	Yes
Kidney cancer		Yes	Yes
Bladder cancer		Avoid – tumours can be oestrogen sensitive	Yes
Cervical cancer	All	Yes	Yes

Type of cancer	Subtype/ risk group	HRT recommendation	Vaginal oestrogen
Endometrial	Low and intermediate risk	Yes	Yes
	High–intermediate risk	Discuss and individualise benefits/risks with specialist	Discuss and individualise benefits/risks with specialist
	High risk: ER/ PR negative	Discuss and individualise benefits/risks with specialist	Discuss and individualise benefits/risks with specialist
	High risk: ER/ PR positive	Avoid	Discuss and individualise benefits/risks with specialist
	Advanced and metastatic	Avoid	Discuss and individualise benefits/risks with specialist
Uterine sarcoma	Leiomyosarcoma	Avoid	Avoid
	Endometrial stroll sarcoma	Avoid	Avoid
Colorectal cancer		Yes	Yes
Vaginal cancer		Yes	Yes

Type of cancer	Subtype/ risk group	HRT recommendation	Vaginal oestrogen
Vulval cancer		Yes	Yes
Ovarian cancer Fallopian tube Primary peritoneal	High-grade serous	Discuss and individualise benefits/risks with specialist	Yes
	Low-grade serous stage 1	Discuss and individualise benefits/risks with specialist	Yes
	Low-grade serous stage 2+	Avoid	Discuss and individualise benefits/risks with specialist
	Endometrioid stage 1	Yes	Yes
	Endometrioid stage 2+	Discuss and individualise benefits/risks with specialist	Yes
	Clear cell	Yes	Yes
	Mucinous	Yes	Yes
	Granulosa cell stage 1	Discuss and individualise benefits/risks with specialist	Yes

Type of cancer	Subtype/ risk group	HRT recommendation	Vaginal oestrogen
Ovarian cancer Fallopian tube Primary peritoneal	Granulosa cell stage 2+	Avoid	Yes
	Germ cell	Yes	Yes
	Borderline tumour: no residual disease	Yes	Yes
	Borderline tumour: peritoneal implants, micro invasive disease, residual disease, recurrence	Discuss and individualise benefits/risks with specialist	Yes
Blood cancers (leukaemia, lymphoma and myeloma)		Yes	Yes

Note that when we say, 'Discuss and individualise benefits/risks with a specialist,' it's because there isn't always strong, reliable evidence on the safety of hormone replacement therapy after certain types of cancer. This can make prescribing it more complicated. In cases where the data isn't clear, both you and your doctor may need to acknowledge some uncertainty and work together to decide the best way forward.

For those of you who have learned that HRT is possible after your particular type of cancer, there are still additional considerations to keep in mind. Your health is multifaceted and there is so much to consider when weighing up the risks versus benefits of taking HRT. If you also have an autoimmune disease or a blood-clotting condition, for example, this needs to be taken into consideration. However, we know that early menopause can negatively impact your bone density, heart health and metabolic functions, and timely hormone replacement is essential to mitigate these risks. So do get the ball rolling and speak to a doctor about it.

HRT After Breast Cancer

Although the use of HRT after cancer is rarely straightforward, it becomes even more complex after certain types, particularly breast cancer. Some women, despite their diagnosis and being told HRT is not suitable for them, still want to understand their unique risks and benefits. In most cases, this is because their menopausal symptoms are impacting their everyday life, or they are concerned about the potential negative impact of early menopause on their long-term health. While some find doctors willing to discuss this with them, many feel they have nowhere to turn.

I have met women who want to know what their risks and benefits are 15 or even 20 years on from the completion of their cancer treatment. Others want to know during treatment, as they struggle so much without the HRT that they had to come off as soon as they were diagnosed with cancer. I've spoken to some women who had had a non-invasive form of breast cancer (DCIS), while others were diagnosed with more aggressive but non-hormonal types such as triple-negative breast cancers. I have met women at all stages of breast cancer, and all different types. Some were curious about using systemic HRT, some were taking it already, while others wanted more details on testosterone therapy alone. However, everyone currently seems to be lumped together under the same guidance, which is 'one-size-fits-all'. My aim in this chapter is to explore the available evidence so that we can understand why this is a controversial topic and why medical opinions may divide. Let's start by looking at what the international guidelines tell us.

Official guidance and advice

The UK's NICE guidelines on early and locally advanced breast cancer[29] state that women should be informed about the possibility of early menopause and menopausal symptoms associated with breast cancer treatment; they advise that systemic HRT should be stopped in women who are diagnosed with breast cancer; that HRT should not be routinely offered to women with menopausal symptoms and a history of breast cancer; and that HRT is contraindicated in women with a history of breast cancer.

The guidelines then go on to state that, in exceptional circumstances, HRT could be offered to women with severe menopausal symptoms and a history of breast cancer after a discussion about the associated risks.

The Menopause Society advises that systemic hormone therapy is not recommended for survivors of breast cancer. However, if symptoms of oestrogen deficiency are severe and unresponsive to non-hormonal options, women, in consultation with their oncologists, may choose hormone therapy after being fully informed about the risks and benefits.[30]

Between the time when I was preparing for my own menopause and today, a lot has changed. Back then I could not find many people who talked about the use of HRT after breast cancer at all. Recently however, I have hosted a series of workshops with over 180 participants from around the world. Women were eager to connect to others to openly speak about their thought processes, concerns and hopes, and we got oncologists, patients and menopause specialists involved in this conversation too.

What I do know for certain is that:

- Some women with a history of breast cancer are curious and want to know if HRT could help them with their quality of life and long-term health; they want to understand their unique risks and benefits.

- Most women feel they have nowhere to go with their questions and are often being denied even a conversation about HRT.

The first person I came across who spoke about taking HRT after breast cancer was BBC broadcaster Kirsty Lang. In an interview with Liz Earle,[31] Kirsty, who was diagnosed with breast cancer at the age of 53, said, 'The first thing my surgeon said to me was, "You need to stop taking your HRT now because the hormones will act like a fertiliser on the cancer cells."' She stopped taking her HRT and was propelled back into what she called a 'miserable menopause experience'. She had surgery and radiotherapy, and was then prescribed letrozole, a drug to treat hormone receptor-positive breast cancer. Kirsty went on to explain that, like so many other people, she experienced very stiff joints as a side effect of the letrozole, so after two years she switched to tamoxifen, which suited her better. She had also been suffering from terrible hot flushes and night sweats ever since she stopped HRT. Initially she assumed that, because of her cancer, going back on HRT was not an option, but she then came across information that challenged this narrative. She explained how she consulted a gynaecologist and expert on menopause, and asked if she should take HRT, and the specialist said, 'It's all about your attitude to risk'. Kirsty then started to take HRT, and, after some tweaking, it helped reduce her hot flushes, helped with her mood and anxiety, and she was also sleeping better.

When I first heard Kirsty's story, I was mainly confused, because I had always assumed that HRT after breast cancer was not an option. But my interest was piqued because her story showed me that experts' opinions on this topic are divided. Some practitioners will give a hard 'no' and won't even discuss the topic with their patients; others, like the one Kirsty found, give you an option and look at making a decision based on your individual risks.

This spurred me on to listen a little bit more closely to other women's stories, and I went on to speak to many of the prescribing doctors. My mind was blown by the intricate situation I was uncovering. It was far more detailed than just answering the question of whether HRT after breast cancer is safe – it involved understanding individual circumstances, needs and risks in a much more nuanced way.

The Impact of HRT on Breast Cancer Recurrence and Survival

Is HRT safe after breast cancer? This is where it gets complicated. The standard response is that there is not enough evidence to provide a definitive answer, but I know you might be wanting to know a little more, so let's delve deeper. To gain expert insights, I sat down with Mr Vikram Talaulikar; Dr Laila Agrawal, a medical oncologist and haematologist specialising in breast cancer treatment in the US; and Professor Richard Simcock, a consultant clinical oncologist in the UK, alongside some other experts.

Mr Talaulikar explained, 'Sometimes opposing views arise about whether a woman should consider HRT after breast cancer. This stems from a lack of robust evidence about the use of modern safer forms of HRT following breast cancer, as studies on hormone replacement therapy after a breast cancer diagnosis are limited and some have faced criticism. As a result, opinions remain divided, with some supporting HRT on an individual basis and others firmly against it.' He went on, 'What happens when you try to give hormones back after a breast cancer diagnosis? That's the question. Because of course that would be a good solution to counteract the many symptoms of the menopause and it would also impact long-term bone and heart health, for example. This of course has to be balanced against the risk of recurrence of cancer and overall mortality.'

To fully understand the development of research, Dr Agrawal took us back to the early 1990s. 'A number of retrospective observational studies were published looking at women who used HRT after breast cancer. Many of these studies showed no increased risk of recurrence or mortality in women who took HRT. This really set the stage to start the first randomised control trial (RCT) where this could be evaluated more rigorously.'

What's important for us to understand is that observational studies are different from RCTs. Since they are not randomised, the underlying risks of the groups may be very different. For example, women at lower risk of breast cancer recurrence might be more likely to choose hormone therapy than those at high risk. RCTs, which are considered the 'gold standard' in terms of reliability, involve creating two groups: one receives the treatment (like HRT) and the other gets a placebo or alternative treatment. Researchers then compare the outcomes between the groups over time to determine effectiveness and safety. 'Both types of studies are important but have different strengths and limitations,' Dr Agrawal explained.

She continued, 'The first RCT that investigated the safety of hormone replacement therapy for breast cancer survivors was the HABITS study. It started enrolling in 1997 [32]. There were about 434 people randomised, including some on medications like tamoxifen and aromatase inhibitors. After about two years, though, the study was stopped early due to an increased number of breast cancer recurrences in the women selected for the hormone replacement therapy arm. At that time there were 26 recurrences in the hormone therapy users compared to 7 in the non-users. This meant that the hormone therapy users were 3.3 times more likely to experience a cancer recurrence. The difference was due to local recurrence, meaning another tumour was found in the breast, or in the other breast (contralateral), but it had not spread to other parts of the body (metastatic disease). Later on, the extended follow-up reported that 39 women in the hormone therapy arm had a recurrence compared to 17 in the non-user group. That means that hormone therapy users were more than twice as likely to have a new cancer event.

'The second randomised control study was the Stockholm trial, which was conducted between 1997 and 2004. It too aimed to evaluate the safety of hormone replacement therapy in breast cancer survivors, and it included about 378 women, but in this study they wanted to minimise the use of progestogen.[33] They also had more women who were taking tamoxifen, which has an oestrogen-blocker effect in the breast. But when the HABITS trial closed early, the investigators of the Stockholm trial decided to terminate their trial early too. In contrast to the HABITS trial, there was no increased risk of cancer recurrence noted in the hormone therapy users. The extended 10-year follow-up also showed no increased risk of cancer recurrence. As both trials were closed early, we just cannot draw firm conclusions.'

The third trial is called LIBERATE. Dr Agrawal said, 'LIBERATE was a trial that evaluated tibolone. Tibolone is a synthetic hormone that mimics the effects of oestrogen, progesterone and testosterone. This trial was different to the HABITS trial and the Stockholm study as it used a different hormone. Tibolone is not approved in the US, but is available in other parts of the world. At the time they thought tibolone was a good candidate as an acceptable option for HRT after breast cancer, but this trial showed an overall increased risk of recurrence in the people assigned to use it. After a three-year follow-up with over 3,000 patients enrolled, they found 15.2 per cent of people had a recurrence in the tibolone arm and 10.7 per cent had a recurrence in the placebo group, with most recurrences being metastatic disease. Here, the conclusions are clear: tibolone should not be used after a breast cancer diagnosis.'

Let's look at some other factors that contribute to making this a complicated subject. Mr Talaulikar explains, 'One of the criticisms of the HABITS study, which showed an increased risk of recurrence, is that some of the hormones that were used as part of the HRT were synthetic progestogens given in very high doses. Women today would be prescribed much lower doses and other safer types. Additionally, we are talking about tiny, tiny numbers of study participants compared to the millions and millions of women who will be diagnosed with breast cancer and be treated over the next 10, 20, 30 years. One of the biggest issues though is that the study was terminated after two years and so we can't make conclusions about the long-term safety of HRT as we just don't know. One could criticise that the small amount of imperfect data is now being extrapolated to stop millions of women from accessing hormone replacement therapy. But nevertheless, this data is what we go by and what has informed the guidelines.'

Moving forward without robust data

Knowing that the best data we have is over twenty years old, mainly from trials that used older forms of HRT and were terminated prematurely, can leave many people feeling at a loss. What does all of this mean for me?, you might ask. In my quest to find out more, I was fortunate enough to have a conversation with Professor Richard Simcock of University Hospitals Sussex NHS Foundation Trust. He is also the charity Macmillan's chief medical officer. As someone who is particularly interested in patient communication and shared decision-making, he was the best person to explain. 'We have women struggle with the symptoms of treatment-induced menopause and we have doctors perplexed at how best to help them. It's understandable that women might want to know if HRT could help them. First of all, we have to accept our ignorance. Let's assume that we don't get a new randomised control trial that tells us that HRT is safe after breast cancer. So we will always be carrying some uncertainty. As an observer and a participant in this debate, I think one of the issues is who carries the uncertainty? Whose risk is it to prescribe HRT to a patient? Some doctors may take a slightly more paternalistic view because they think the risk is theirs as the prescriber. I believe that if there is a risk, that risk is held by the person taking the drug. What we need to do is have a shared decision-making space, where, as carefully as we possibly can, we convey to the person receiving the drug that there's uncertainty and ensure they understand this.'

'The challenge we face is determining by how much HRT might increase the risk of breast cancer recurrence for an individual,' Professor Simcock continued. He went on to echo what the other doctors I have spoken to also said. 'The HABITS study is over twenty years old and we know it has several limitations. But let's say you accept this bad data, as it is the best data we have, as a worst-case scenario. It indicated that HRT could increase the risk of breast cancer recurrence about threefold. We then need to work out what an individual's risk of recurrence is after their treatment. To illustrate, let's assume someone's risk of recurrence after all their cancer treatment is 4 per cent. According to the HABITS study, if the patient then takes HRT, this risk could theoretically triple, increasing it to a potential 12 per cent. This is simply an example to guide the conversation and support the patient in making an informed decision about their care. It allows for an educated, adult-to-adult discussion about whether they are willing to accept that potential risk in exchange for the benefits that HRT might bring them. To me, this is the kind of dialogue we should aim for.'

I am not sure about you and how you feel. Do you feel we are so desperately in need of more research? That it's unfair that the best data we have is bad and old data? And how do you feel about Professor Simcock's way of working out how we could quantify this potential additional risk; should you accept working with the data in question? Some people will want to do everything at all possible to lower their risk of a cancer recurrence. For other people, their symptoms of menopause might be so severe that they are willing to accept an element of uncertainty for the potential benefit of HRT. Everyone I spoke to had different reasons for why they wanted to consider HRT after their breast cancer diagnosis – or, for some, why they would never entertain the thought of taking it. To me, it has always been and is about really listening to the individual, understanding what truly matters to them, and facilitating a neutral conversation.

HRT after triple-negative breast cancer (TNBC)

So what about triple-negative breast cancer, which is non-hormone-receptor-positive? Can patients with a history of TNBC who have gone into early menopause or are experiencing menopausal symptoms receive hormone replacement therapy?

Board-certified medical oncologist Dr Eleonora Teplinsky, based in the US, is an expert in breast and gynaecological cancers. She is a brilliant educator on social media and answered this in one of her posts, so concisely: 'While the data out there is limited, it does *not* suggest harm for menopause hormone therapy (MHT) in patients with triple-negative breast cancer. Two systematic reviews have been published, which summarised and evaluated all of the relevant studies on the use of HRT after hormone-negative breast cancers.[34 35] These analysed the evidence from the multiple studies we have to date and both showed no increase in the risk of breast cancer recurrence for women with hormone receptor-negative tumours who are taking MHT.'

Dr Teplinsky explains that, despite this, some oncologists advise against MHT in triple-negative breast cancer. She explains that the current definition of a triple-negative tumour is one that is oestrogen receptor (ER)- and progesterone receptor (PR)-negative and has a less than 1 per cent ER/PR expression. In other words, if less than 1 per cent of the cancer cells have these hormone receptors, the cancer is classified as a triple-negative tumour. But in the past, a 10 per cent cut-off was used to determine the cancer type. So someone with 9 per cent ER expression who was treated as having TNBC could still have some oestrogen receptor activity – and it is this that raises concern. Additionally, there is concern that a very small percentage of triple-negative breast cancers could recur as oestrogen receptor (ER)-positive cancers.[36] Dr Teplinsky concludes, 'What do I recommend? In general, I am supportive of

MHT use in hormone receptor-negative cancer in those with premature menopause and/or menopausal symptoms after a thorough discussion of the data that exists and the potential concerns and risks/benefits.'

I questioned the lack of robust data when I interviewed renowned breast oncologist Dr Elizabeth Comen from the Memorial Sloan Kettering Cancer Center (MSK) in New York City. Dr Comen, who had just published her fabulous book, *All in Her Head*, said, 'Triple-negative breast cancer patients who have gone through accelerated menopause because of chemotherapy or other causes, or they have to have their ovaries removed because of BRCA or other inherited risk mutations, often want to know if they can use HRT safely. It is very frustrating that there are not enough studies done on those women! The bottom line is, we've abandoned women in medicine and we need to do better.'

Testosterone after breast cancer?

As part of my many conversations with doctors and breast cancer survivors from all over the world, I came across many stories of women enquiring about testosterone therapy alone and whether it would be a 'safer option' after breast cancer. Usually the answer is that, because testosterone can convert into oestrogen in the body, it is not recommended for the use of breast cancer patients. On a podcast episode, I interviewed Dr Rebecca Glaser, a retired US-based breast cancer surgeon who is involved in research on testosterone therapy by pellet implant. Over the last 10 years she has evaluated and treated over 1,500 breast cancer patients. She explained, 'In our research, we look at the administration of testosterone delivered in combination with an aromatase inhibitor (i.e. anastrozole or letrozole) combined in the pellet implant. The aromatase inhibitor stops the conversion of testosterone to oestrogen. The pellets sit beneath the skin in the fatty tissue and can deliver the testosterone and aromatase inhibitor for about three months. Patients report an improved quality of life, fewer menopause symptoms and, most importantly, no increased risk of recurrence was observed to date.' Dr Glaser adds, 'We believe it is the consistent continuous release of testosterone that gives the benefit, alongside the aromatase inhibitor stopping the conversion to oestrogen.'

Although promising, this research is limited because it has not been replicated in other studies. I know a few young breast cancer patients in the UK who have actively explored this option. They worked hard to navigate the healthcare system to find supportive doctors, shared research with their oncologists, and engaged in numerous conversations with various healthcare professionals. Needless to say, as you can imagine, they have invested significant time and energy, and, despite the high cost of private treatment, they have pursued this treatment option. They have kept me updated over the years, and I continue to be inspired by their unwavering determination to find the best path for themselves. I have also met breast cancer patients who were prescribed topical testosterone gel while on, for example, tamoxifen. With each conversation, I became increasingly aware that doctors and patients adopt different approaches and manage risks and uncertainties in many different ways.

A difficult conversation – should it be about patient choice?

The thing that interests me the most when we talk about the use of HRT after breast cancer is having an open conversation. Currently, most women seeking to understand their personal risks and benefits of using HRT are struggling to find a doctor to talk to. I met the lovely Jo, who had endured a really difficult time with menopause after her breast cancer treatment; it left her feeling like a shadow of her former self. She was desperate for relief and did a lot of research into HRT and wanted to explore that as an option. However, during a telephone appointment with her oncologist, the oncologist flatly refused, stating, 'I can't have a conversation with you about it.' So that was the end of it. 'It felt like a real kick in the stomach,' said Jo, and it left her feeling unheard and upset.

Dr Corinne Menn, who I introduced in Chapter 3, brings not only her professional expertise but also personal experience as a 23-year breast cancer survivor. Dr Menn was diagnosed with receptor-positive breast cancer in her twenties while still doing her medical training, and offers a unique perspective on navigating menopause after cancer. She went on to take tamoxifen, and explained to me that she had a myriad of symptoms due to the side effects of the drug, but muddled through the best she could. A few years into treatment she had her ovaries removed. This was not related to her breast cancer treatment but due to a genetic mutation. Of course it triggered immediate surgical menopause. Corinne had many symptoms that came with that. She finished 10 years of tamoxifen, during which time she became a mum, and, after years of suffering from the collateral damage of premature menopause, she did her research and decided that going on a low-dose regime of hormone replacement therapy (HRT) would be the right thing for her. She said, 'We can't throw all breast cancer survivors into the same bag. What we need is a nuanced discussion and a personalised conversation with each patient.'

For years I have been having conversations with women where I really try to understand what makes them tick. I want to understand their deepest concerns and, with each conversation, I learn something new. Many of the HRT-after-breast-cancer chats were a little less open and a little more 'hush-hush' than my usual conversations, as if it wasn't quite right to enquire about it. But we must. Because those of us who enquire push boundaries. It shows our doctors that we really do need help in how to manage menopause after cancer. And as I have said before, this will, in return, improve research and inform science – for all of us. So to all of our sisters who were brave enough to do what they felt was important to them, thank you.

It is not lost on me that it will most likely prove to be a challenge if you would like to discuss HRT after breast cancer with someone in the medical profession. You need to find a clinician who is open to discussing your concerns and hopes with you, and willing to engage in shared decision-making with you. And I hope doctors will commit to learning how to communicate effectively and engage in these important conversations with their patients.

Sally Kum, Breast Cancer Now's Associate Director of Nursing and Health Information, with whom I have had numerous conversations over the years, is passionate about communication. She often says to me, 'It's all just about learning to communicate with one another.' And I completely agree. Decision-making can be very challenging when we have to work with data that is anything but perfect. Let's remember that your values, preferences and priorities are important when making difficult medical decisions. I often say, I am not here to support opinions, but to support each individual I work with. I feel it should always be your choice and decision how you want to live your life and manage your risks.

HRT After Gynaecological Cancers

For a long time, I believed that the uncertainty about using HRT after cancer was primarily an issue for those affected by breast cancer. However, it was through working, a few years ago, with Dawn, who had been diagnosed with endometrial cancer, that I realised the gynaecological cancer community faces many of the same challenges as the breast cancer community. Dawn is a resourceful, diligent and reflective person who was willing to put much effort into her quest to find out whether HRT was right for her. It took her a long time, and conversations with several doctors, to find the information she needed to make an informed decision. Mr Vikram Talaulikar of University College London confirms, 'As with breast cancer, data about the use of systemic HRT following treatment of various gynaecological cancers is limited. In some situations, the lack of robust evidence makes decision-making difficult for patients and healthcare professionals, creating challenges in assessing risks and benefits. The good news is that we've got more and more data in the last five to ten years. We are now able to offer hormone replacement therapy (HRT) after individualised discussions to a wider range of patients with different gynaecological tumour types and stages, tailoring treatment to each person's unique situation. In some cancer types, the evidence for the safety of HRT is lacking robust data and, of course, we always have to take into consideration each patient as an individual. That's when a specialist and patient need to discuss the individual situation and decide together what is the right thing to do.' He acknowledges, 'The long-term effects of cancer treatments, such as menopause, often go overlooked. There is usually no dedicated support for managing these late effects, and women may be left to navigate this on their own, without referrals to specialist clinics.'

Please refer to the table on pages 105–108 for details of when HRT is considered safe following various types of gynaecological cancers. These guidelines align with the new (August 2024) recommendations from the British Gynaecological Cancer Society and the British Menopause Society, which provide comprehensive information for healthcare professionals managing menopausal symptoms in women treated for gynaecological cancer. You can download their guidance document from the internet for more detailed information – I have linked it in your digital handbook for you too.

Vaginal/Topical Oestrogen

Vaginal oestrogen is a topical, local oestrogen therapy used to treat the genito-urinary syndrome of menopause (GSM). GSM results from a decline in oestrogen levels and encompasses a large variety of symptoms that include vaginal dryness, irritation or burning, painful intercourse, itching, vaginal discharge, a reduction in vaginal elasticity, frequent urination, urgency, painful urination and urinary tract infections. I talk about this a lot throughout the book as it is such a common and, in some cases, debilitating condition for many women, but particularly for cancer survivors after all types of cancer. For most cancer survivors, vaginal oestrogen is a safe and effective treatment, with a few exceptions that I will address below. Unlike systemic hormone replacement therapy, which affects the whole body, vaginal oestrogen is applied directly to the vaginal and vulval tissues in the form of creams, pessaries, tablets or rings, targeting local symptoms with minimal to no absorption into the bloodstream.

Dr Alison Macbeth, who I introduced you to earlier in the book, has established a dedicated menopause clinic for breast cancer patients, after recognising the significant need for specialist menopause care for cancer survivors. We have run many sexual-health workshops for cancer survivors together and Dr Macbeth is passionate to educate; she says, 'I see so many cancer patients struggling with horrendous GSM symptoms, which can come on quite suddenly during or after cancer treatment. We have oestrogen receptors all over the body, including in the vagina, vulva, bladder, urethra and pelvic floor. As oestrogen levels decline, the vaginal tissues lose elasticity and become more fragile, and dryness increases. This can make arousal more difficult, and changes in vaginal pH can disrupt the vagina's microbiome, leading to a rise in urinary tract infections. Bladder function is also often affected, resulting in increased urgency and frequency.' Dr Macbeth adds, 'Some women don't want to admit they're struggling – it can be embarrassing to talk about symptoms to do with your vulva, vagina or loss of libido – but it's crucial that they do.'

GSM symptoms do not improve on their own over time, so, regardless of what type of cancer and cancer treatment you have had, get the ball rolling and ask for some help.

Talk about your symptoms

According to an article by ASCO (American Society of Clinical Oncology), sexual dysfunction, although prevalent among cancer survivors, is rarely addressed.[37] The article references a survey of cancer survivors that found that nearly 9 out of 10 respondents reported some change after cancer treatment that negatively impacted their sexual health, yet few survivors were warned about this potential side effect, and even fewer were formally asked about their sexual health after treatment. What's more, results showed that women who survive cancer may be significantly less likely than men to have their sexual side effects addressed by their provider. Based on these findings, the authors of the study recommended that oncology practices integrate questionnaires that assess sexual health as part of survivorship care for all patients.[38]

Because so many women suffer from severe symptoms and, with the right strategies, help is available, I believe every female cancer patient should receive basic sexual-health education, including information on skin-safe vaginal moisturisers, lubricants (more on pages 80–83), the option of vaginal dilators and the facts about vaginal oestrogen.

The section below is courtesy of Dr Alison Macbeth, who, alongside her expertise as a doctor, is also a determined campaigner advocating for increased support and access to sexual health services for cancer survivors. Her commitment to improving holistic care for survivors is both inspiring and essential.

What you need to know about vaginal oestrogen

Vaginal oestrogen is a low-dose treatment, designed to target the tissues in the vaginal, vulval and urinary area. You can choose from different products depending on preference, and sometimes you might have to try a few options to see what works best. It can take a few weeks to feel a really good improvement in symptoms, and it's important for you to persevere before you change to a different product. Using vaginal oestrogen can be transformative for women with GSM symptoms, and in most cases symptoms do very much improve in a short period of time.

- You can use different treatments together, such as an oestrogen pessary and a cream, for example. This can help with symptoms on the outside (vulval area) and the inside (vagina).

- Vaginal oestrogen can be used alone or alongside systemic HRT.

- Ask your doctor if you don't see the improvements you want. You can try different products; different things suit different people.

- Don't stop your treatment when symptoms improve, or they will come back. Symptoms are also likely to return if, as many women say they do, you continue using your vaginal oestrogen when symptoms improve but become a little less regimented about it.

- Skin-safe vaginal moisturisers and lubes (see pages 128 and also 296–297) can be used alongside vaginal oestrogen; it's not a one-or-the-other decision!

- In women who have not had breast cancer, vaginal oestrogen is not associated with an increased risk of breast cancer and you do not need progesterone to go with it.[39]

- The effect of using vaginal oestrogen for a whole year is the same as that of one to two systemic HRT tablets, so there is a big difference between the two.

- Vaginal oestrogen does not increase the risk of dying of breast cancer in those who have had breast cancer.

Types of local vaginal oestrogen

There are two types of vaginal oestrogen: Estradiol (E2) and Estriol (E3). Estriol is shorter-acting and lower-dose (about ⅛ of the dose of vaginal Estradiol).[40]

Pessary

Pessaries are inserted into the vagina, generally using an applicator. There are different types. Imvaggis is one, containing Estriol. Imvaggis pessaries are small, waxy and bullet shaped. Unlike other pessaries, Imvaggis doesn't come with a plastic applicator and is designed to be inserted with your finger, which reduces plastic waste.

Cream or gel

Ovestin is a cream and Blissel is a gel. These contain Estriol and are inserted into the vagina with an applicator. The cream can also be applied externally to your vulva.

Ring

A soft flexible silicone ring containing estradiol that you can insert into the vagina. The product is called Estring and it releases a slow and steady dose of oestradiol over 90 days into your vagina. It only needs to be replaced every three months. You can leave the ring in position to have sex.

Tablets

Vagifem, Vagirux and Gina all contain the same 10mcg estradiol tablet for vaginal use, which comes as a tiny tablet in a plastic inserter. Vagifem comes with pre-filled applicators, which makes it convenient to use but less eco-friendly. Vagirux, on the other hand, comes with reusable applicators. It's better for the enviroment but some people find it a bit fiddly to use. Gina is the over-the-counter version of Vagifem. All three work the same way – just different packaging and applicator options.

In the past few years two new treatments have also become available, which function slightly differently to the above – vaginal pessaries of DHEA (dehydroepiandrosterone) and oral ospemifene (selective oestrogen receptor modulator). Since these are newer treatments, not all international guidelines currently consider them safe to use after some cancers as long-term evidence is not yet available.

Official guidance on use of local oestrogen after breast cancer

While there is often uncertainty and concern in the cancer community about the use of vaginal oestrogen, particularly for those undergoing active breast cancer treatment, it's important to know that the conversation is more nuanced than it may seem. Just as with systemic HRT, I've consulted with leading doctors in the field to provide you with the latest information, so you can make well-informed decisions about your options. Together, we'll explore current guidelines, and I will also share with you the latest evidence to help clarify when and how vaginal oestrogen can be used safely. I hope this will empower you to feel confident in your choices.

While the general approach to managing GSM in breast cancer survivors is similar worldwide, different guidelines have slightly different recommendations for treatment options:

- Both the British Menopause Society (BMS) and the Menopause Society in the US suggest vaginal oestrogen for breast cancer survivors with genito-urinary symptoms if non-hormonal vaginal moisturisers do not provide relief. They note that low-dose vaginal oestrogen is an effective treatment, with minimal absorption into the bloodstream.

- For those on active treatment for hormone receptor-positive breast cancer, the BMS advises that vaginal oestrogen can be used by women taking tamoxifen but not those on aromatase inhibitors. In contrast, the American College of Obstetricians and Gynecologists (ACOG) advises that those on aromatase inhibitors can use low-dose vaginal oestrogen after discussing the risks and benefits with their doctor.

- If vaginal oestrogen is not suitable, the ACOG guidelines recommend considering vaginal DHEA or oral ospemifene as an alternative option. However, the BMS notes there isn't enough long-term data on the safety of ospemifene and DHEA.

- When discussing the various consensus statements, it is also important to consider the St Gallen International Consensus Statements (2023), which state that vaginal oestrogen can be considered for women on aromatase inhibitors to alleviate symptoms of GSM, particularly when symptoms are unresponsive to moisturisers and lubricants.[41]

Latest evidence on the safe use of vaginal oestrogen for breast cancer survivors

I've heard countless stories from breast cancer survivors whose oncologists and surgeons have approved vaginal oestrogen, with many of them reporting huge relief from their symptoms. Some even describe it as life-changing. Unfortunately, at every workshop we still hear from women suffering from severe symptoms, who have been told by their doctors that they cannot use vaginal oestrogen. Dr Alison Macbeth echoes this: 'I see women every day who have been denied vaginal oestrogen despite significant symptoms that not only severely impact their quality of life but also prevent them from exercising and having sex, and wake them up multiple times during the night to urinate. This lack of sleep can lead to brain fog and over time to weight gain, depression and relationship issues. Women's joint pain gets worse due to the inability to stay active. It becomes a downward spiral. Recurring UTIs can lead to urosepsis, antibiotic resistance, and even kidney injury from repeated antibiotic use.' She goes on, 'Vaginal oestrogen is safe to use in previous breast cancer survivors whether they had a hormone-sensitive positive or negative cancer and it is safe to use in patients on tamoxifen. Where the waters get a bit muddy is in hormone-sensitive breast cancer patients who are currently on treatment with aromatase inhibitor medication. These women are often told to switch to tamoxifen or just get on with vaginal moisturisers, which in many cases will not be enough to manage symptoms. Many women stop their endocrine therapy altogether because of unmanaged GSM symptoms. The trial often quoted when women are denied the use of vaginal oestrogen while on aromatase inhibitors is the Danish study, published in 2022.[42] However, the data collected for this study dates back to a study from 1997 to 2004 and breast cancer treatments and the formulations of vaginal oestrogen have moved on a lot since then.[43] There are many things one can criticise about the study, but, to keep it simple, even the dosages of vaginal oestradiol used were much higher than what we would prescribe today. The ultra-low-dose oestriol (Imvaggis and Blissel), which I now regularly prescribe to all my breast cancer patients, wasn't even available back then.' Dr Macbeth is keen to add, 'This study is often the one used by oncologists to deny women on aromatase inhibitors the use of vaginal oestrogen. By understanding these limitations and presenting this information to their oncologists, patients can open up a more nuanced and evidence-informed discussion about their options.'

US-based oncologist Dr Eleonora Teplinsky who is also a brilliant educator about sexual-health issues for cancer survivors, writes, 'There remains so much controversy about vaginal oestrogen and breast cancer risk of recurrence and survival. The systemic absorption of vaginal oestrogen is minimal, but some doctors still remain hesitant. A study published in *Jama Network Oncology* examined the impact of vaginal oestrogen on breast cancer survival.[44] They looked at nearly 50,000 females from Scotland and Wales. In vaginal oestrogen users compared to non-users, there was no evidence of a higher risk of breast cancer-specific mortality for those with hormone-positive cancers, even in those on aromatase inhibitors. This is great news! Additionally, a new study published in November 2024 in the *American Journal of Obstetrics and Gynecology* looked at the association between vaginal oestrogen use and breast cancer recurrence.[45] The authors found eight studies that met their criteria. Six studies looked at breast cancer recurrence in the context of treating the genito-urinary syndrome of menopause with vaginal oestrogen and found NO association between vaginal oestrogen use and increased recurrence risk. There was also NO increased risk of breast-cancer-specific mortality with the use of vaginal oestrogen.'

In 2023, Mr Talaulikar and a colleague conducted their own research to find out if using vaginal oestrogen could increase the risk of breast cancer recurrence among survivors; and they also wanted to see if these treatments raised oestrogen levels in the blood. Their findings were published in the *Sage Journals*.[46] Mr Talaulikar explained, 'After searching the literature, we found none of the trials reported an increase in breast cancer recurrence. Additionally, we found no significant or lasting increase in blood oestrogen levels after using these vaginal oestrogen products or low-dose vaginal DHEA gel. To better understand the long-term risk of breast cancer recurrence in survivors using these treatments, we now need more trials over longer periods of time using the modern low-dose vaginal oestrogen preparations.'

To conclude, if you struggle with ongoing GSM symptoms since your breast cancer diagnosis, and you have tried non-hormonal options such as vaginal moisturisers and lubricants and are still experiencing issues, make sure to speak to your doctor and advocate for yourself. If your medical team has not felt comfortable prescribing vaginal oestrogen, show them the studies we have referenced above – or seek a second opinion!

I have also linked the studies in your digital handbook to accompany this book, allowing you to share them with your doctor. These resources can help ensure that your doctor stays up to date with the latest information.

Vaginal oestrogen for gynaecological cancer survivors

Mr Talaulikar is passionate about ensuring that all women are adequately counselled on their options for vaginal oestrogen after gynaecological cancer, ideally even before treatment begins, so they can make informed decisions and receive timely support for managing GSM symptoms. He explains:

> *'Vaginal oestrogen can offer significant benefits in alleviating GSM symptoms for patients after gynaecological cancers, but we must consider specific aspects, such as time since diagnosis, type of tumour and type of treatment that has been had. Most low-dose commonly used vaginal oestrogen products are associated with no or minimal absorption of oestrogen into systemic circulation. However, in cases of oestrogen-sensitive tumours, when genito-urinary symptoms do not respond to first-line non-hormonal options, treatment decisions about vaginal oestrogen need to be individualised. In many situations, the relief of GSM symptoms and quality of life will take priority for women, and vaginal oestrogen can be prescribed following discussion about limitations of current evidence and potential risks versus benefits.*
>
> *'Because so many patients experience severe genito-urinary syndrome of menopause (GSM) following treatment for gynaecological cancer, it often feels like, by the time they reach me as a menopause specialist, they have already endured*

significant discomfort for a long time. Ideally, I would like to see these women before they undergo cancer treatment or surgery. Having a thorough pre-operative plan and discussing what to expect can help minimise delays in accessing support post-treatment and empower women to take an active role in managing their care.'

I hope the information here gives you a solid understanding of what is currently happening in the world of vaginal oestrogen. I recognise that everyone comes with their own suitcase full of symptoms and their own specific advice from their doctor. I also want to remind you that you don't have to suffer in silence. If your symptoms are affecting your quality of life, please seek support and explore all your options. Ask your doctor to discuss with you the latest evidence on vaginal oestrogen for your specific situation; and it is okay to get a second opinion too! There is help available, and you deserve to feel your best. As you move forward, remember that you have the power to advocate for yourself. Stay informed, ask questions, and don't be afraid to seek out specialists who understand the complexities of menopause after cancer.

REFLECTIONS

Take a few moments to reflect...

1. Have you learned something new about hormone therapy after cancer?
2. How do you feel at the lack of robust data? And given the data, do you feel a conversation about HRT or local oestrogen therapy for yourself is what might be next for you?
3. Are you clearer about the use of vaginal oestrogen and the safety of it for most cancer survivors?

POSITIVE ACTIONS

1. Track your GSM symptoms using the table on pages 34–35 and ensure you speak to your doctor should you need help – speak up about what you are experiencing.
2. Get the ball rolling and speak to your medical team should you want to enquire about hormonal treatment options.
3. Keep speaking up about your experience of menopause after cancer so that your story can drive research, new medication and a better future for all survivors.

CHAPTER 7
HOW TO MANAGE CHEMICAL MENOPAUSE CAUSED BY ENDOCRINE THERAPY

If you are taking drugs like tamoxifen, aromatase inhibitors or medications that suppress ovarian function, you may experience menopause symptoms. These medications, also often referred to as endocrine therapy, are an important part of cancer treatment; they stop the effect of oestrogen on breast cancer cells, doing so in different ways.

As many of you will know and experience, these drugs can come with significant side effects, which can be particularly challenging, as symptoms of oestrogen deficiency like hot flushes, joint pain, fatigue, genito-urinary symptoms and emotional changes can be intense and difficult to manage. Plus, many women have to embark on these treatments for five to ten years. This is a long time and, if you are struggling, you may feel there is no end in sight. If you're on endocrine therapy because your breast cancer has come back or spread, or if you have been diagnosed with metastatic disease, you'll usually continue taking it for as long as it is effective.

In this chapter, I aim to give you lots of practical tips for managing your side effects. With the help of Dr Claire Macaulay, a highly respected breast oncologist at the Beatson West of Scotland Cancer Centre, I will provide information, strategies and support to help you stay on your treatment for as long as possible while minimising its side effects.

Alternatively, this knowledge can empower you to have informed conversations with your doctor about your options. I will also address the emotional challenges that often accompany long-term cancer treatment, as well as include a list of contraindications that are frequently asked about.

Which Cancers Are Treated with Endocrine Therapy?

Several cancers can be hormone receptor-positive, meaning their cells have specific receptors on their surface – proteins that bind to hormones circulating in the body, such as oestrogen and progesterone. Determining the hormone receptor status of your cancer (together with the grading and staging) helps your medical team work out the best course of treatment for you. Breast cancer is the most common example. About 80 per cent of all breast cancers are oestrogen receptor-positive or 'ER-positive'.[47] About 65 per cent of these are also progesterone receptor-positive or 'PR-positive'. When hormones bind to these receptors, they activate signalling pathways that promote cell growth and division.

Ovarian and endometrial (uterine) cancers can also be hormone-sensitive, especially certain subtypes that are affected by hormonal changes. While less common, cervical cancer may in certain situations be influenced by hormonal factors. If your cancer has a significant number of receptors for either oestrogen or progesterone, it's considered hormone receptor-positive. Tumours that are ER-positive or PR-positive are more likely to respond to endocrine therapy than those that are ER-negative or PR-negative.

After I finished my own active cancer treatment, which included surgeries, chemotherapy and radiotherapy, my doctor told me that, because of the type of cancer I had (triple-negative breast cancer), I would not be offered endocrine therapy as my tumour did not respond to it. I remember feeling very scared about that information, because I felt there was nothing else my cancer team could do to help keep my cancer at bay and stop it from recurring. Back then, I had no idea of just how much impact different endocrine treatments could have on women. For many, the end of active cancer treatment is a difficult period, bringing with it a whirlwind of mixed emotions. There's often little guidance on how to navigate life post-treatment, leaving many feeling that they are expected just to move forward without much support. While friends and family are most likely wanting to celebrate the end of active treatment with you, the reality is that you might be managing ongoing endocrine therapy, the effects of which not many people understand. Yet, the thousands of people in our groups and the many women I have spoken to have shared that dealing with the side effects of endocrine therapy is often the most challenging part of their cancer journey.

The Most Common Endocrine Therapy Drugs

Tamoxifen is used to treat oestrogen-positive breast cancer and belongs to a class of drugs called selective oestrogen receptor modulators (SERMs). Tamoxifen blocks the effects of oestrogen on ER-positive breast cancer cells. Tamoxifen does not cause menopause but it may cause you to feel the symptoms that are associated with it. Tamoxifen is used to treat breast cancer in both premenopausal women and postmenopausal women.

The other medication category is called aromatase inhibitors (AIs).[48] Before the menopause, oestrogen is mainly produced in the ovaries. After the menopause, the ovaries no longer produce oestrogen, but some oestrogen is still made in body fat. This process involves an enzyme (a type of protein) called aromatase. Aromatase inhibitors stop this enzyme from working. Basically, AIs strip the body of all oestrogen. They include anastrozole, exemestane and letrozole. AIs are often used in postmenopausal women, but they can also be used in premenopausal women in combination with drugs to stop the ovaries from working, or if the ovaries have been removed.

Goserelin (Zoladex) and leuprorelin (Prostap) are types of hormone or endocrine therapies commonly used in the treatment of breast cancer. They are commonly used for premenopausal women to suppress oestrogen production, sometimes during chemotherapy to preserve fertility.

Fulvestrant (Faslodex) is a selective oestrogen receptor degrader (SERD) typically prescribed for postmenopausal women.

Side effects of endocrine therapy

The benefits of endocrine therapy can vary significantly from person to person, as can its side effects. Endocrine therapy can help reduce the risk of breast cancer coming back or spreading, so finding ways to manage those common side effects is key to getting the most out of these medications and is why it's essential that we dig into this topic. Currently, women in our community who are prescribed these treatments express three major concerns:

- Lack of preparation: many women report feeling unprepared when starting the medication, saying they were not informed that their treatment might trigger significant menopausal symptoms.

- Lack of acknowledgement of symptoms: many patients say they raise their symptoms with their doctors, but don't feel understood in relation to how much their symptoms impact their life.

- Lack of support with symptoms: most people say they have no idea where to turn to for support.

Even though we get hundreds of comments on our posts about endocrine therapy, the same few themes come up over and over again.

> *'My doctor said just to take this little white pill (tamoxifen) every day for ten years and that most women are fine on it; they don't have problems.'*

> *'Nobody said that exemestane would come with these crippling side effects. I can't even walk without pain.'*

> *'I was sent off with the tablets with little discussion. My oncologist said not to believe all these women in the Facebook group when I expressed concern over possible side effects!'*

> *'I had intense side effects in the first year. My oncologist completely dismissed my concerns.'*

> *'I stopped my medication and never told my doctor – she would just have argued with me and I had no energy for the fight.'*

'Tamoxifen made me feel suicidal.'

'I feel as if I am 90 years old, I'm only 42!'

I could fill a whole book with stories of how these therapies impact people's quality of life. They range from those who have heard from others about how much they struggle as a result of taking the medication, and are so worried that they never start the treatment in the first place, to those who stop their medication early because the side effects become too overwhelming. There are women who get to the end of their treatment without too many symptoms; however, we hear fewer of those stories. And that's normal. When people are okay they may not feel a strong need to share their experiences online. But almost all say that they feel very much alone in navigating this chapter of their cancer treatment, and the majority feel very unsupported.

Before we dive into this topic, I want to remind you to focus on your own experience. It's easy to get caught up in all the negative stories about side effects, but your journey with these medications is yours alone. While it's good to be informed and to know what to do if you experience side effects, try not to compare yourself to others – what happens to someone else won't necessarily happen to you.

Dr Macaulay says, 'Depending on your type of cancer, your age and many other factors such as grade of cancer and stage at diagnosis, your medical team will work out which endocrine therapy will work best for you. Both tamoxifen and aromatase inhibitors can come with side effects and you may experience some of them or many of them to varying degrees. Please remember, not everyone struggles in the same way!'

Tamoxifen side effects include hot flushes, night sweats, fatigue and vaginal dryness. Fluid retention, irregular periods or loss of periods, nausea, fatigue, weight gain and headaches are also very common. Long-term and less common side effects from tamoxifen include blood clots, deep vein thrombosis, liver issues and endometrial cancer. In premenopausal women, tamoxifen can cause the thinning of your bones. By comparison, in postmenopausal women, tamoxifen has an oestrogen-like effect on bone tissue, helping maintain bone density.

Aromatase inhibitors (AIs) come with similar side effects to tamoxifen, but because they strip the body of all oestrogen, side effects can feel more severe. Joint pain can be a particularly difficult problem, as well as vaginal dryness and the other symptoms associated with GSM (genito-urinary syndrome of menopause). Other side effects of AIs include thinning or weakening of the bones (osteopenia and osteoporosis) and high cholesterol.

Why endocrine therapy can be challenging

Many women come to our workshops and say they are worried about starting their tamoxifen or AI medication. They have read horror stories online about the potential effects and are worried they're going to experience the same debilitating symptoms. Dr Claire Macaulay explains the facts: 'We know that between 20–25 per cent of people will never actually start the medicine that they're given. As an oncologist, I can't predict which side effects you might experience from treatment. You could have some, none or all of them. But just because there's a long list of potential side effects, it doesn't mean you'll experience any or all of them – and, if you do, we can try and find ways to manage them.'

Some women choose not to start endocrine therapy, and for those I've spoken with who made this decision it was always after extensive research and careful consideration. It can be incredibly challenging to go against medical advice, but it's essential to feel empowered to make the choice that feels right for you. Everyone has a unique perspective on weighing up risks and benefits, and, once we have all the information needed to make an informed decision, it's important to trust our own judgement and do what feels best for our individual health.

> *'I thought long and hard about starting endocrine therapy and had lots of discussions with my medical team, but in the end decided not to take it as my overall benefit of taking it was so small. In my case it was less than 2 per cent. I felt it was about understanding the risk of recurrence and the benefit of the drugs.'* ***Susanna***

Compliance rates for adjuvant endocrine therapy in hormone receptor-positive breast cancer is really challenging.[49] They are at around 60 per cent after five years,[50] so somewhere between one-third and half of people won't complete the course of endocrine therapy because of the side effects. That's a really big issue worldwide, because the benefit that the treatment could have is being lost,' explains Dr Claire Macaulay. Dr Alison Macbeth, who, like Macaulay, sees so many breast cancer patients in her menopause breast speciality clinic, agrees: 'I see so many women who have just stopped their treatment themselves after feeling so horrendous. We know compliance on endocrine medications really drops off after the first six months. It is really difficult for breast cancer patients – as soon as they are over their acute treatments they are discharged by oncology and then have only virtual follow-ups by the breast units in the form of an annual mammogram, and most no longer get physically seen for follow-up. So it's no surprise these women feel they have nowhere to turn to when struggling with the side effects of endocrine therapy.

> *'I made the decision to stop after five years (instead of the recommended ten) and then went onto monthly Zoladex injections to switch ovaries off before eventually opting for a bilateral oophorectomy and coming off drugs altogether. It's been a heck of a journey and lots of research and reading and talking to people to reach all of those decisions. Crucially, I took my time with each decision and waited until I was confident in the decision I made before acting on it.'* **Vicky**

When I spoke about the issue of compliance rates with breast cancer survivor and menopause specialist and OBGYN, Dr Corinne Menn, she told me: 'Most patients are suffering the side effects of their endocrine treatment and want to quit it, but don't understand its benefit. And some women are suffering with the side effects of endocrine therapy and want to stay on it but have no idea that their actual benefit is really so small.'

Understanding your individual benefit

If you're struggling with side effects from your endocrine therapy and are starting to wonder whether it is worth continuing with it, it might be helpful to understand the true benefit of your treatment. You may not have had a full discussion with your doctors when you started the therapy, or you may not want to talk about numbers and statistics as this can be scary and unsettling. But if you think knowing could help you make a decision about what to do, it's never too late to go back to your doctors and ask. Whether you've been on endocrine therapy for a while, or are just about to begin and are unsure of the exact benefits for you, don't hesitate to reach out to your medical team for clarification. Remember, you're never a bother – your health and peace of mind are important!

A way to establish what the benefit of endocrine therapy is to you is to consult the Predict tool, which your oncologist can explain to you.

In the UK, this is an algorithm-based tool that can be used by doctors and patients to see how different treatments for invasive breast cancer might improve survival rates after surgery. It is based on thousands of studies and data from women with breast cancer about what happens to people in the long term. Oncologists use it to determine what treatment they are going to offer their patients. They input specific details about the patient's cancer diagnosis, including information such as age, tumour size, grade, lymph node involvement, hormone receptor status, HER2 status, and the type of surgery or other treatments being considered. The tool then uses statistical models based on the historical data, which help estimate the benefits of various treatments and the overall prognosis. The tool also predicts the potential benefits of additional treatments such as chemotherapy, hormone therapy and other interventions, which can help patients and doctors make more informed decisions about the best course of action.

Dr Macaulay explains, 'It's really important that individuals understand what benefit they are getting from the treatment they've been offered. Some patients will have a 1 per cent additional survival benefit at ten years after diagnosis, and for some other patients the benefit will be much greater. Survival benefit means, out of a hundred people who take treatment, how many extra people will be alive because of it. So a 1 per cent survival benefit at ten years means that for every hundred people who take the treatment, one extra person will be alive ten years later. For some people, a 2 per cent additional survival benefit may be worth it, for someone else it may not. It is a complex dance between impact on quality of life now from side effects, and reducing the risk of cancer coming back later on. We all have individual views about managing risk and what side effects are worth that risk or not. Some women will handle their treatment without needing detailed information, preferring to get through it and move on. Some will want to understand the full picture.'

I remember one lady sending us a message after a workshop with Dr Macaulay. She wrote, 'Dani, you won't believe it. After listening to the oncologist on your workshop I plucked up the courage and asked my own oncologist to talk me through my benefits of being on tamoxifen. By that point I was actually feeling suicidal, I was feeling so low. The oncologist said my benefit was only 1 per cent! In my eyes, there was no point me being on the treatment, and I am upset that I was not told this before!'

I think this is a really good example as it teaches us quite a few things:

- It highlights how crucial it is for patients to feel empowered to ask questions about their treatment options and understand the potential benefits and risks involved. This way we can make more informed decisions about our health and treatments.

- It reminds us that we all process information differently at different times. Some people want to know all the facts from day 1. Others find that all too much and prefer information being drip-fed to them over time. It is hard for your doctor to know which type of person you are. Ultimately, for me, this emphasises the significance of patient advocacy and asking the questions when you are ready!

- Most importantly, each person is different, and the benefits of endocrine therapy will vary from one person to another. Some of you reading this will be able to ponder over what to do, while others, with a secondary cancer diagnosis for example, will have far fewer options.

If you'd like to see how the Predict tool works and get a more detailed explanation about it, then we have a couple of YouTube videos on our channel in which Dr Claire Macaulay explains it. The link is in your digital handbook.

Were you adequately prepared for the challenges?

A common problem I see is that people are not adequately prepared for what may happen to them during endocrine treatment, therefore their expectations of it are not realistic. Some people think that once their active cancer treatment is 'done' they're now 'only' on endocrine treatment. I believe this narrative needs challenging. It implies that you should have fewer side effects and less support and that you should just get on with it. Family, friends and colleagues might also think you're 'done' with cancer, and over time it might become harder to explain that, in fact, you're still on treatment that can have a daily impact. In fact, you've embarked on an endurance ultra-marathon and, just like any athlete, you need strategies and support to get through it. In my opinion, it starts with providing more information to patients and an open conversation and a dialogue between you and your doctor.

It is my hope that, if all parties involved, patients and doctors, continue to raise awareness of the difficulty with endocrine therapy, advancements within research, science and the pharma industry will look towards creating medication with fewer side effects or coming up with better strategies to combat the ones we currently experience. We know that patient-reported symptoms play a crucial role in advancing medical science and pharmaceutical development. We've seen this process lead to positive change in other areas of medicine. Take rosiglitazone, a drug used for Type 2 diabetes. Over time, patients and healthcare providers reported cardiovascular issues, including an increased risk of heart attacks. These reports led to large-scale studies and new research, resulting in safer and more effective alternatives for controlling blood sugar, which had a more favourable impact on heart health. As of recent estimates, about 2.3 million women globally were diagnosed with breast cancer in 2020, according to the World Health Organization (WHO),[51] and a large proportion of these will be offered long-term endocrine treatment; this, in my opinion, is enough people who can drive change for better care. So please don't think you have to suffer in silence. Speak up and share your experiences! The least that will happen is that someone else in a similar situation feels less alone. In the best-case scenario, our stories will shape research and drug manufacturing, leading to treatments with fewer side effects, and improving the lives of millions of other cancer survivors.

Tips to manage endocrine treatment when you are experiencing side effects

In this section, I'll share practical tips for managing the side effects of endocrine treatments. These insights come from workshops I've hosted with doctors, as well as valuable advice shared by members of our community who have found these strategies effective. Oncologist Dr Claire Macaulay says, 'Small tweaks can make a big difference. For many people, the side effects of treatment can improve over time, often easing after the first three to six months and within the first year.'

Consider discussing the strategies highlighted on the following pages with your healthcare team should you experience stubborn symptoms. And remember, the information throughout the rest of the book will hopefully give you many tips on easing menopause symptoms holistically. For example, see pages 291–295 in Chapter 11 to discover how movement can help with joint aches, or learn about which non-hormonal options can help manage hot flushes in Chapter 5.

Tamoxifen tips

- Some people may benefit from splitting the dose of tamoxifen. Once a day is easier to take as you only have to remember it once, but some people may find their symptoms improve if the dose is halved, so they take half in the morning and half in the afternoon.

- Taking tamoxifen at night can be helpful if you experience nausea. For most people, nausea wears off after they've been on it for a few weeks. Taking it at night-time can also help if you have joint pain that you find gets worse towards the end of the day.

- If you are really struggling, ask your team about the possibility of a drug holiday. Stopping tamoxifen for 12 weeks to see if symptoms ease off can help you understand if it is the medication causing them. If it is, then you can discuss strategies to help going forward. If your symptoms don't ease off, then you will know it is not the medication. In some cases, this can help you decide whether to stay on the medication or not.

- Some people agree with their oncologists that they will take half the daily dose (10mg instead of 20mg), take it every other day, or take it for 9 months out of 12. We don't have a clear consensus yet about whether that impacts long-term outcomes as trials are still ongoing, but it's worth speaking to your doctor to discuss this if you're really struggling; together with your doctor, you may decide some protection is better than no protection.

- For some people particular brands of the medication have fewer side effects than others, for example on your skin or joints. There are no large studies to support this, but there is plenty of anecdotal evidence. It's good to keep a symptom diary and be more aware of how different brands can potentially affect you differently. Some women feel a difference within a couple of weeks. In the UK, GPs can prescribe specific branded tamoxifen or specific manufacturers and then make a note of your chosen brand on your repeat prescription. And your pharmacist can also request certain brands or provide you with an alternative that will work best for you. It's still the same medication, so it will give you the same benefit. One lady told me, 'Different brands can definitely make a huge difference. They switched me to a different one a few months ago, which caused my feet to hurt so much that I had to buy new shoes and it impacted my activity levels. Since then, I am trying to work out which brands have the least side effects, with the help of the pharmacist.' Another said, 'It took me about nine months of trying different brands to find the one that suited me – I don't have any joint pains with the one I'm taking at the moment and I would be in tears walking with another. My pharmacist said it's the filler in the medication, not just the drug itself.' I know it can be hard to access the brand that suits you best, but it's worth giving it a go.

- Another woman told me, 'The first few months on tamoxifen were horrible – I had an allergic reaction on my face and neck, suffered really badly with sweats and hot flushes, and I couldn't sleep. I'm happy to report that with diet, exercise and the help of venlafaxine (medication prescribed for hot flushes) I'm feeling all better. Very rarely have I got hot flushes now.' (See pages 75–76 and 78–79 to learn more about non-hormonal medication for hot flushes.)

Aromatase inhibitor tips

- All three aromatase inhibitor drugs (letrozole, anastrozole and exemestane) have similar effects and no one drug is better than another, but some people may get on better with a particular one.

- Each AI is made by a number of different manufacturers. Some of the tablets may have different additional ingredients (for example preservatives). This does not change the effectiveness of the treatment. Try figuring out if a certain brand of the same drug suits you better. It is worth asking to be prescribed a different brand .

- Just like with tamoxifen, you can try to unpick which side effects are being caused by the medicine and what isn't the fault of the medicine. The best way to do this is by talking to your doctor and discussing whether to stop the treatment for four to six weeks to see. Most people will know within this time whether they are better off without the treatment or not. If you feel your symptoms very much improve when you're off the treatment, however, then your doctor may be able to switch you to a different type of endocrine therapy to try.

- If you are not a great deal better off the drug than you were on it, then discuss what lifestyle changes could be looked at, and what other medicines or approaches you might be able to add in that might help you with your side effects, such as the ones outlined throughout this book.

Switching Between Different Types of Endocrine Therapy

Many people are switched from tamoxifen to AIs or the other way round. This choice will largely depend on your symptoms, which will be balanced against the benefit the medication can give you. For instance, tamoxifen is less likely to cause joint pain compared to aromatase inhibitors. This is why filling in a symptom checker is so important. Have a detailed conversation with your team. They can explain to you what the difference in benefit is for you personally on each of the treatments. The difference may be very small. If switching from one to another gives you an improved quality of life and hence allows you to stay on treatment, this may be a good strategy for you.

Don't think it's a 'take or leave it' type situation. Look at all the medical non-hormonal treatments, complementary therapies and lifestyle changes outlined in this book to help support you and to help you manage the menopausal side effects you are experiencing.

> *'I tried anastrazole for six months and the joint pain and stiffness were too much to continue with. The breast care nurse is changing my drugs to exemestane. I have had the tablets for six weeks and not had the courage to start them, but I will. The view of the nurse was to give it another go as not everyone has the same side effects on the different drugs. If I do, however, she said we could still try tamoxifen in the future.'* **Suzie**

Contraindications at a glance[52]

Often, women who I speak to wonder what to eat and what supplements they can take to help them manage the symptoms of menopause. And often they feel confused and worried about possible interactions between their medication and supplements or foods. Any medication may have contraindications when combined with supplements, certain foods, herbal medication or complementary therapies, but with tamoxifen there seems to be a particularly long list.[53] That's because for tamoxifen to be effective your body must convert it into its active form, endoxifen. This conversion involves multiple steps, each requiring a specific liver enzyme – a protein that accelerates cellular processes. Certain foods, drinks and medications can interfere with the enzyme's ability to convert tamoxifen to endoxifen, to varying degrees. Below is an at-a-glance guide to some of the contraindications for tamoxifen, but please do your research too and speak to your doctor.

Possible contraindications when taking tamoxifen

- Grapefruit and grapefruit juice can reduce the effect of tamoxifen treatment.

- Turmeric and curcumin in concentrated supplement form should be avoided – in cooking it's fine.

- Black cohosh is currently contraindicated (see page 172), though more research is being conducted and needed.

- St John's Wort is to be avoided.

- Asian ginseng is to be avoided.

- Antidepressants, such as fluoxetine, paroxetine and sertraline, have the ability to reduce the effectiveness of tamoxifen – your doctor will know which ones to prescribe instead.

- Using blood thinners requires careful medical supervision, as tamoxifen can increase the risk of blood clots, and doctors need to balance clot prevention with bleeding risks.

Possible contraindications when taking AIs

Luckily, the list of contraindications while on AIs is not so long, but please always check with your doctor before adding a new supplement.

- Grapefruit and grapefruit juice can reduce the efficacy of the treatment.

- It is worth noting that alcohol should be avoided or limited while taking aromatase inhibitors, as alcohol consumption may decrease the efficacy of this medication.[54]

- They can interact with other medications such as some anti-epilectic medications, some heart medications and specialised antibiotics.[55]

Stopping Endocrine Therapy

Stopping endocrine therapy, whether in agreement with your doctor or not, is never an easy decision to make. But many women simply feel that they can't carry on coping with the side effects they are experiencing – the impact on their life is just too great. This conflict can evoke a wide range of emotions, making your decision process intensely challenging. And I wish everyone had more support and more opportunity to mull it over with a doctor.

Oncologist Dr Macaulay says 'Some women stop the treatment and pretend they are taking it and never tell their doctor. Mixed feelings of guilt and shame play a big part here and many say they don't want to feel like they're going against medical advice or setting themselves up for a confrontation with their oncologist. It shouldn't be like that – this is a partnership. What's important is that the decision is made in conjunction and in partnership with your healthcare team.'

The Emotional Complexity of Navigating Endocrine Treatment

If you are reading this right now, and you are somewhere along the decision-making process of what to do about your endocrine therapy, I want to acknowledge just how hard this can be. From the hundreds of conversations I have had with women, I have learned that you may feel it's impossible to know what might be the right thing to do for you. You might feel you can't carry on like you are right now, and you are hoping for relief, but at the same time you are scared of what the future might hold. The uncertainty can be incredibly hard to sit with. All I can offer is: try to speak with your doctors, learn about your own benefits for the drugs you have been prescribed and take your time in making a decision that is right for you. Our emotions, combined with the facts, play a crucial role in shaping our decision-making process. Besides, you might find yourself grappling with a whirlwind of mixed emotions – sometimes even opposing feelings – all at once. It's perplexing, yet it's a deeply human experience. Below I list some examples of strong emotions that come into play, many of which I have experienced myself time after time; perhaps some of them resonate with you too?

Fear: *One of the most overwhelming emotions I encounter. The thought of stopping treatment and the worry about an increased* *risk of cancer recurrence can be paralysing, making it difficult to think clearly and make decisions.*

Hope and despair: *The hope for a longer, healthier life through continued treatment is powerful. However, when side effects severely impact daily life, this hope can quickly turn to despair. The constant struggle to balance quality of life with the hope of extended survival can make you feel pretty hopeless and frustrated.*

Guilt and responsibility: *Many of the women I speak to feel a deep sense of responsibility towards their loved ones and themselves. The decision to stop treatment can be accompanied by guilt; patients might feel they are letting down their families or not doing everything possible to fight the disease.*

Relief and doubt: *For some, the decision to stop treatment may bring an initial sense of relief from the burdensome side effects. However, this relief can be quickly overshadowed by doubt and second-guessing. Patients may constantly question whether they made the right choice.*

It's essential to honour that this can be a really hard and ongoing situation to manage, and that it may take a long time to decide what to do next or where to turn to for help. I hope this section, and indeed the whole book, will give you oodles of inspiration on how to look after yourself and how to manage the symptoms caused by your chemical menopause.

REFLECTIONS

Take a few moments to reflect...

1. How much do you think your current treatment is impacting your everyday life? In which ways? Fill in the symptom checker on pages 30–32.
2. Have you reached out to your doctor already, or have you spoken to the specialist nurse and asked for help?
3. Have you already tried some of the strategies outlined in this chapter?

POSITIVE ACTIONS

1. Speak to someone in your medical team and enquire how they can support you with the treatment you are on.
2. Would you want to know your true benefit of being on the treatment you have been prescribed? If so, ask one of your doctors to explain it to you.
3. Acknowledge that the treatment you are on is not 'just a little white pill'. If you're struggling, that's normal – give yourself a big pat on the back! You're amazing!

CHAPTER 8
COMPLEMENTARY THERAPIES

In my many years of navigating life as a cancer survivor and in early menopause, I have asked myself often, 'Could mindfulness really help my anxiety?', 'What herbal remedy might help joint ache?' and 'Is collagen safe after cancer?' And I'm not alone. Researchers at Cancer Research UK estimate that 30–40 per cent of people with cancer use complementary and alternative medicine (CAM).[56] I believe the number to be much higher, because I've hardly met with another cancer survivor who has not thought of adding supportive therapies to their toolbox, in the hope to recover, heal and support how they are feeling. In our community, there are countless daily discussions about complementary therapies. From supplements to mindfulness, there's no topic left untouched.

The term complementary therapies can mean different things to different people, so I want to be clear about what I understand it to mean. For me, they are the therapies used *alongside* your conventional treatments: acupuncture, yoga, meditation, dietary supplements and herbal medication, massage, CBT (cognitive behavioural therapy), CBT-I (cognitive behavioural therapy for insomnia), hypnotherapy, counselling and therapy.

Integrating complementary therapies into your routine can make a profound difference to you and your life by helping to improve your menopause symptoms after cancer. 'The evidence around the value of "integrative oncology" (which is the definition of what we are doing in integrating complementary approaches into our standard cancer care) in terms of improving outcomes for people with cancer is overwhelming and cannot be ignored,' writes Dr Nina Fuller-Shavel, a leading integrative medicine doctor, author and educator, who also has extensive education in nutrition, integrative and functional medicine, herbal medicine, Traditional Chinese Medicine, yoga and mindfulness. Yet few hospitals are able to offer referrals to complementary services.

The situation is different in different countries, however. Having been raised in Austria, I know that European health services include complementary therapies in their standard cancer treatment plan more frequently and, in fact, in all their healthcare. My dad, who has suffered with addiction disorder and mental health issues for nearly two decades, and who has regularly had to spend time in hospital, is always offered complementary therapies such as yoga, physical activity and cold-water treatments to promote his health and wellbeing alongside his comprehensive treatment plan. I'm also able to get herbal medicine and special creams for my chronic lymphoedema prescribed by doctors in Austria, or I can buy them at pharmacies there, which is not the case in the UK. Some can be purchased online, but that means there is no consultation, which is obviously not ideal. In my opinion, and in an ideal world, we would give all cancer patients access to an integrative medicine doctor who could help them put together a personalised plan. But we know that cancer survivorship care is not always ideal. Everywhere I look, most people tell me they are navigating this entire aspect of their care and recovery very much on their own, muddling through somehow.

Perhaps you too are piecing together different strategies, using a bit of a hit-and-miss approach? I was the same. I remember the countless sleepless nights I spent scouring the internet for information on alternative therapy options and strategies, desperately seeking ways to improve my wellbeing and my menopausal symptoms. In those early days, I really had no idea what I was doing and why; I lacked strategy and a plan, which resulted in a cupboard overflowing with supplements and a sense of confusion and overwhelm.

Yet, amidst the chaos of supplement research and experimentation with different therapies, I found a glimmer of hope: a sense of empowerment in taking charge of my health journey. I felt good that I was doing something to be proactive. Dr Fuller-Shavel and her co-author Dr Penny Kechagioglou write in their book *Integrative Oncology in Breast Cancer Care*, 'There is a sense of control and empowerment when patients make the decision to use integrative oncology approaches, although the dangers of unregulated use is sometimes underestimated by patients.'

In this chapter I'll be exploring the empowering array of options available to you, shedding some light on any contraindications and offering guidance on where to find further information. You could fill several books with discussions of these important strategies, so I've chosen to focus on the practices or dietary supplements that have the most evidence supporting their effectiveness (and there is plenty), plus the ones that are more frequently discussed in our community. For example, we have lots of discussions about acupuncture, but far fewer about reflexology or reiki. The reason I want to go into quite some detail with this chapter is that adding complementary therapies to your routine can not only help you reduce your menopause symptoms and those from your cancer treatment, as well as help you with your emotional trauma;

it can also help you stay on your long-term cancer treatment, such as endocrine therapy, which in turn can help improve survival rates.

Think of an actual toolbox. It may contain a hammer, a screwdriver, some nuts and bolts, a spirit level, nails, Rawlplugs and maybe even some of those picture-hanging sticky tapes. You decide whether to take out a hammer and a nail to hang your picture or use the sticky tapes, or perhaps you might even need a screw if it's a heavier picture you're trying to hang. That's exactly what we do with this chapter. You can tap into tools such as acupuncture, CBT or herbal medication to help with anxiety, for example, but often you'll need to use a variety of complementary therapies and approaches to give you the best outcome. Not every tool will work for everyone, and there may be tools that have helped you that I have not referenced in this book. Keep doing what works for you! What matters most is understanding the options available to you and taking the time to assess and reflect on what feels right for you. As you go through this chapter, keep the following important questions in mind:

What resonates with you?

What are you drawn to?

What have you tried?

What are you curious about?

And do you even have the energy right now to get your head around any of this?

I truly believe there is a right and a wrong time to add any new strategy to our lives. Sometimes, we are just so full up, so tired, so busy, so 'all over the place' that we are best to do less, not more. And I'll show you how to do that in this chapter too. I had the privilege of speaking with Dr Shelly Latte-Naor, an experienced integrative medicine doctor who works at the prestigious Memorial Sloan Kettering Cancer Center in New York, known for its large complementary medicine department, which offers various integrative therapies to support cancer patients. Dr Latte-Naor shared a valuable piece of advice: 'I always remind patients that they don't have to take on everything that is out there, as this can lead to a self-care burden. Instead, it's important to curate interventions that truly fit into their lives.'

Below are some of the most commonly discussed and evidence-based complementary therapies, which can help with your menopause symptoms. Always consult with your healthcare team before starting any complementary treatments.

Acupuncture

Acupuncture is commonly used to alleviate pain, reduce stress, promote relaxation and address a variety of health conditions. It has been practised for thousands of years and is rooted in Traditional Chinese Medicine. By inserting thin needles into specific points on the body, the practitioner can stimulate nerves, muscles and connective tissue, which can prompt the body to release various biochemicals, such as endorphins, your body's natural painkillers. Acupuncture is also believed to influence levels of the neurotransmitters serotonin and dopamine, which regulate mood, pain perception and bodily functions. Out of all the complementary therapies, acupuncture is one of the most well-known approaches, and helps to alleviate symptoms such as hot flushes, stress, anxiety, depression and sleep disturbances, all commonly associated with conditions like menopause, chronic pain and cancer treatment.

'Acupuncture works for me in reducing hot flushes and improving sleep/ mood, and totally relaxes me. It also helped with the emotional fallout after the medical treatment ended, but it took a while to find a good therapist,' writes one member of our Facebook group; and others, who say much the same thing, add that their oncologist has referred them for it. We will talk about access and cost later on. For now, let's look at the evidence for its benefits.

Dr Latte-Naor explains, 'Acupuncture is mentioned in at least five of the National Comprehensive Cancer Network (NCCN) guidelines for symptoms management in cancer survivorship and in the ASCO-endorsed guidelines of the Society for Integrative Oncology[57] for use in aromatase-inhibitor-related joint pain.'[58]

A 2024 analysis of randomised trials[59] that looked at the use of acupuncture in women undergoing endocrine therapy for hormone receptor-positive breast cancer found that acupuncture significantly reduced hot flushes and other endocrine symptoms such as night sweats. In fact, 64 per cent of participants saw at least a 50 per cent reduction in hot flush scores, with the benefits lasting up to 10 weeks after treatment. These improvements also helped patients stick to their prescribed endocrine treatment, potentially reducing the risk of recurrence and improving long-term outcomes for breast cancer survivors.

For me, this is what it's all about – how can we find strategies and enable women to better deal with some of the so very harsh menopausal symptoms that come as a result of cancer treatment? Whether you are on endocrine therapy, or navigating menopause symptoms years after active treatment, I know how many of you think you have limited treatment options. So finding access to complementary therapies such as acupuncture may be a good next step for you.

How can you access it?

Cost and finding the time to attend the appointments are hurdles to receiving a treatment such as acupuncture. If you are still being seen by an oncologist or cancer nurse, don't hesitate to enquire with your team and ask for a referral or recommendation. Some will be able to refer you to an acupuncturist, but in other parts of the country and world you will have to find a therapist yourself. If you go and look for an acupuncturist yourself, choose someone who has experience working with cancer patients or who has received specialised training in oncology acupuncture. They should understand the unique needs and challenges faced by individuals undergoing cancer treatment. Always consult with your healthcare team before starting any complementary treatments, including acupuncture.

In the UK, charities are also a good starting point. Wonderful places, like Future Dreams House in London, provide group ear acupuncture sessions for free, which many people I know find really beneficial for relaxation and symptom relief.

For those averse to needles, seed acupuncture or auricular acupuncture is also an option. It involves placing tiny seeds or beads on specific acupuncture points on the ear. These are held in place with a little tape and you stimulate the points yourself by pressing on the seeds. Take some time to research what your local cancer charities offer, as they may provide acupuncture as part of their services.

Herbal Medication/Supplements

There are many plant extracts that can help ease an array of menopause symptoms. But I have not yet met many cancer survivors who were not scratching their heads at the long list of potential herbal supplements, confused about what might help them or might not. The herbal medicine landscape is vast. I have spoken to people who don't believe that there is much benefit to using herbal medicine, or they're just not drawn to trying it. Others want to try it but are unsure what type is best for the symptoms they have. And some worry that there are contraindications to an existing medication or cancer treatment they're on. And then there are those who are unsure because of the type of cancer they have had, usually a hormone-sensitive cancer. That's a lot to unpack.

But if herbal medication and supplements are potent enough to interfere with medication in a negative way – as it's important to point out – it logically follows that they are also potent enough to offer substantial benefits. While cynics may focus on the potential downsides, I believe it's important to recognise the positive possibilities as well. Because these add to the options that we so very much need.

But what I feel we need to address right at the start is, where do we get herbal medicine from? What type should you buy? And how can you make sure you are buying good-quality products? In a pretty much unregulated supplement market, it is helpful to follow some practical steps to ensure you can access herbal supplements in a safe and effective way.

In an ideal world, and if you can afford it, I would suggest seeking help from a medical herbalist, who will get to know you as a whole person and gather your full and comprehensive medical history, including your medication details and treatment regime. This way, you wouldn't have to worry about any contraindications or the safety of a product, or doing any research of your own.

Often, diet, sleep and digestion are thoroughly discussed alongside your symptoms and what you need support with and, of course your medical herbalist will contact your oncologist or cancer team if anything needs discussing. In many cases you will get a herbal medicine prescription, consisting of various herbs or a tincture targeting your specific symptoms. Often this is sent out to you by the medical herbalist. As you can see, this is a very different process to buying a herbal remedy over the counter.

The National Institute of Medical Herbalists is the main governing body for herbal practitioners in the UK. The 'Find a Herbalist' section of its website enables you to find a registered practitioner in your area. If you want to get the most out of herbal medication and you can afford to see a medical herbalist, then I believe this is the best way to go about it. Most importantly, if you do go down this route, contact the herbalist first and ask about their experience of working with people with a history of cancer.

Of course I know not everyone has the option of seeking the help of a medical herbalist. So if you decide to do your own research into herbal supplements, here's what to look out for before you decide which supplement is right for you:

- Choose products with the THR logo: Traditional Herbal Registration; this is granted by the Medicines and Healthcare products Regulatory Agency (MHRA). This means the medicine complies with quality standards relating to safety and manufacturing, and includes instructions on how and when to use it.[60]

- If you are undergoing active treatment, it is important to inform your oncologist if you are starting any herbal medicines as they can interact with cancer treatments like chemotherapy, radiation or hormone therapy. If you are no longer in active treatment, it's still a good idea to speak to your medical team or your pharmacist, as they can guide you on safe options, assess potential interactions with any ongoing medications, and help you make informed decisions about your health.

- The Memorial Sloan Kettering Cancer Center website (www.mskcc.org) offers an excellent tool for checking herb–drug interactions. Simply enter the herb you're researching, and the tool provides detailed information on potential benefits, side effects and possible contraindications with other medications you may be taking.

Most resources on menopause that address herbal medication state that there is a lack of long-term data, or that evidence is sparse and the information provided is limited. Some might argue that there are fewer randomised control trials (RCTs) on herbal medications compared to conventional drugs due to factors like limited funding from pharmaceutical companies, as herbal remedies often can't be patented.

At the same time, millions of cancer survivors are seeking ways to manage their menopause symptoms, often after being told they cannot use HRT, which leads many to explore herbal remedies for relief. Add to this the fact that the menopause market is flooded with herbal supplements designed for women without a history of cancer, and you may be left wondering which, if any, might be suitable or helpful for your situation. I have chosen the following herbal supplements because they are the ones that most commonly come up in questions in our community and have been suggested as helpful by some of the wonderful medical herbalists I have worked with over the years. We will explore current guidance on specific herbs, how they may help with certain menopause symptoms, and what potential contraindications to be aware of based on the type of cancer you have had.

The decision to try a herbal medication or supplement is a very personal one. The number-one main mistake I see people make when it comes to choosing a herbal supplement is that they are unclear *why* they are doing so. So ask yourself this question first. Why do you want to explore supplements? Is it to help alleviate a symptom? Or to support your future health? Knowing this will make your research much easier.

Phytoestrogens

There is a lot of confusion around phytoestrogens, and the same questions and concerns from our community come up time and again. Comments like, 'My cancer was hormone sensitive and so my nurse said I can't have anything with oestrogen in it at all, so sadly no soy for me!' or, 'Can I have red clover; I had breast cancer?' are very common.

But when we are discussing phytoestrogens, it's really important to clarify the difference between phytoestrogens found in food and those in supplement form. Phytoestrogens in food are naturally occurring compounds found in plant-based sources, while phytoestrogens in supplements are often concentrated forms that can deliver a more potent dose, potentially leading to different impacts on our bodies. In this section of the book, I will focus on phytoestrogens as supplements, while you can refer to pages 261–263 for information about phytoestrogens in food.

Because phytoestrogens have oestrogenic effects in the body, they can be very useful in supporting menopausal symptoms. There is plenty of research[61] showing their health benefits, from reducing hot flushes, night sweats and mood swings all the way to improving bone health.

In supplement form, phytoestrogens are typically derived from isoflavones and lignans. Isoflavones are the most common source and they can be found in soya and red clover *(Trifolium pratense)*.

The second most abundant class, lignans, are mainly present in flaxseed, although whole grains, vegetables and tea are also sources. Sage *(Salvia officinalis)*, contains other types of phytoestrogens and bioactive compounds, such as certain types of flavonoids used to manage menopausal symptoms due to its ability to reduce excessive sweating and hot flushes. Its oestrogenic effects are slightly weaker than those of isoflavone-rich plants.

Many of the 'menopause supplements' on the market today will most likely contain concentrated forms of some of these phytoestrogens.

Current guidance states that women who have or have had hormone-sensitive cancers, including breast and some types of gynaecological cancers, should avoid phytoestrogens in supplement form (though not in food).

Over the past few years, I've had numerous conversations with Melinda McDougall, a medical herbalist specialising in menopause support. She has played an important role in helping me and many women in our community navigate the complexities of herbal medicine, empowering us to make informed choices. She explains that there has been a long-standing belief that phytoestrogens in supplement form may increase breast cancer recurrence for those with hormone-sensitive cancers, hence the current guidance. She explains that there are two types of oestrogen receptors: alpha and beta receptors. When we talk about hormone-receptor-positive breast cancer, we mainly refer to the alpha receptors that play a role in driving the cancer. Initially, it was believed that phytoestrogens stimulated the alpha receptors, potentially increasing the risk of breast cancer recurrence. However, according to Melinda, current research is debunking this theory. Specifically, new studies are showing that phytoestrogens have a higher affinity for binding to beta receptors, meaning that they may be beneficial for women recovering from breast cancer and reduce recurrence.[62]

'Groundbreaking research trials in this area are being undertaken that may change the shape of this conversation in the future,' Melinda explains. 'Dr Roberta Brinton, who is an internationally recognised leader in Alzheimer's research, has received millions of dollars to study isolated components of soy and red clover,[63] called PhytoSERMs (Selective Oestrogen Beta Receptor Modulator), which contain three phytoestrogens, examining their impact on the female brain and their ability to relieve symptoms such as hot flushes.'[64] In addition, she says they may also have the potential to actually reduce breast cancer risk. It is an ever-changing landscape, with new research and data always coming in, so it's important to keep learning. At the time of writing, Dr Roberta Brinton's research is ongoing; she has not yet published final results.

One of these PhytoSERMs is Femarelle,[65] a type of patented soy extract. I have heard from some women that they have been prescribed these by their menopause specialists to reduce hot flushes and sweats and to help with vaginal dryness, sleep and bone health.

I hope this clarifies what the guidance tells us about phytoestrogens in concentrated form and where we are at with current research. If you have a history of hormone-sensitive cancers and you are interested in exploring concentrated forms of phytoestrogens further, working with a medical herbalist will be your best starting point. Make sure to read Chapter 10, where we talk about the benefit of eating foods rich in phytoestrogen, even for those with a history of hormone-sensitive cancers. There is no need for you to feel you have to miss out!

Other herbal supplements

Black cohosh

Black cohosh *(Actaea racemosa* or *Cimicifuga racemosa)* is used to treat hot flushes and night sweats and reduce menopausal joint pain and anxiety.[66] It was first used by the indigenous North Americans.

'Black cohosh is not considered a phytoestrogen. Early reports suggested it might act like one, leading to caution regarding its use in hormone-sensitive conditions like breast cancer. However, more recent research has shown that black cohosh does not contain oestrogenic compounds,'[67 68] explains Melinda McDougall. Instead, it works through different mechanisms, potentially affecting serotonin receptors, which help alleviate menopausal symptoms such as hot flushes and mood swings without directly influencing oestrogen levels.

It's important to note that current medical guidance advises against taking black cohosh if you've had hormone-sensitive breast cancer and are on tamoxifen.

Melinda also told me that some exciting recent clinical studies have been looking at the use of black cohosh *alongside* tamoxifen.[69] These studies found that black cohosh enhanced the activity of tamoxifen and reduced menopausal symptoms such as joint aches, night sweats, hot flushes and low mood. With this debate in mind, there are calls for additional well-designed clinical studies. As with phytoestrogens in supplement form, if you have a history of hormone-sensitive cancers and you are interested in exploring black cohosh further, working with a medical herbalist will be your best starting point.

Blue skullcap

This is a lesser-known herb, but is one of Melinda's firm favourites. Blue skullcap *(Scutellaria lateriflora)* is a calming and relaxing herb, effective for managing anxiety without being sedative. It can be taken as a tincture or enjoyed as a loose tea. Brewing herbal teas is an easy and inexpensive way of using herbal medicine and people often underestimate the power of it. The hot water extracts the chemicals from the plants and releases them into the water. 'Always try and get loose tea because it's going to be so much stronger and more potent than a teabag. Regularly drinking teas such as blue skullcap three times a day can help reduce anxiety and promote calmness,' Melinda says.

Lemon balm, valerian and passionflower

Melinda says, 'I really enjoy prescribing lemon balm *(Melissa officinalis)* as part of my tinctures – it is an uplifting herb that supports both mood and digestion. It can also be enjoyed as a tea. Valerian *(Valeriana officinalis)* and passionflower *(Passiflora incarnata)* are both effective remedies for sleep, and can be taken as teas, tinctures or supplements – best about half an hour before bed. These plants have no contraindications with hormone-sensitive cancers. You can also use them as teas and enjoy their benefits.'

St John's wort

St John's wort *(Hypericum perforatum)* has been used for centuries to help address mood disorders, light and moderate depression and anxiety, and it often comes up in our conversations. In her book *The Complete Guide to The Menopause*, Dr Annice Mukherjee writes that St John's wort has been studied in large randomised control trials for the treatment of depression, and it has been shown that it is as effective as conventional antidepressants. In terms of menopause, NICE (National Institute for Health and Care Excellence) states that some women have found that St John's wort can reduce their hot flushes and night sweats. However, the ingredients of products containing St John's wort can vary a lot, so, as with all supplements, it's important to buy good-quality products; remember to look out for the THR logo. St John's wort can interfere with a long list of drugs, such as chemotherapy drugs, blood thinners and tamoxifen[70], so always consult your doctor before taking it.

Adaptogens

Adaptogens are plants and mushrooms that help our bodies adapt to stress. They are not among the more traditional plants used for the treatment of menopausal symptoms, like red clover for example, but they are very interesting for cancer survivors to discuss. For one thing, they've become quite popular over the last few years and women sometimes ask me about them. Plus, if you are recovering from cancer or undergoing treatment, your body can be under huge stress. In fact, chronic heightened stress levels are something I feel we all have in common after a cancer diagnosis. Medical herbalist Melinda McDougall explains, 'Adaptogens are remarkable. They can help calm the whole nervous system, help bring down levels of cortisol in the body, which is our stress hormone, and help lower inflammation. There are a variety of adaptogens that may be appropriate for different people and situations.'

Adaptogens have become so popular in recent years that you can find adaptogen coffee brands and adaptogen powders to mix into drinks and smoothies. Some popular adaptogens include ashwagandha, rhodiola and Siberian ginseng, with ashwagandha *(Withania somnifera)*[71] being perhaps the most well-known herbal medicine in the group.

It has become popular among experts and patients for easing symptoms like anxiety and fatigue as well as for improving cognitive function,[72] and we get many questions about it in our community forums. Studies show that it has the potential to improve cancer-related fatigue, in addition to improving quality of life.[73] However, the study authors also say that further study with a larger sample size in a randomised trial is needed to validate their findings.

On my quest to find out more about how we can help our community understand the benefits but also the contraindications to herbal medicine better, and in particular ashwagandha, I met Rebekah Brown, founder of Mpowder, a wholefood supplement brand and community. I shared with Rebekah that so many people, especially those with a history of hormone receptor-positive cancer, are confused about what is a safe product for them and what is not. Rebekah was so moved by the stories I told her that, together with her team of doctors and researchers, she created a brilliant menopause and cancer booklet,[74] which includes links to plenty of studies and particular herbs. You can download it on their website and look at the research yourself.

Rebekah and her team explain that the evidence supporting the use of ashwagandha in cancer care is limited. Although the data so far is promising, much of what has been studied only includes a small number of women. An open-label study with 100 breast cancer patients showed that ashwagandha significantly alleviated chemotherapy-induced fatigue and improved quality of life.

One of Mpowder's doctors, Dr Vera Martins, who holds a PHD in cancer biology, recommends that when purchasing ashwagandha you should be careful to buy the type labelled KSM-66. This is a full-spectrum ashwagandha extract, meaning it's not concentrated or altered.

For years, at every workshop, I have tried to ask medical herbalist Melinda McDougall to suggest a herb for this symptom and another herb for that symptom. But Melinda has frequently and patiently explained to me, 'When you receive a herbal medicine prescription from a trained medical herbalist like myself, you will rarely get just one herb in isolation. Herbs often work synergistically, which means combining different herbs can enhance their effectiveness and balance their effects. For example, one herb might address a primary symptom, while another supports digestion or reduces inflammation, creating a more balanced and comprehensive treatment. This tailored approach is quite different from over-the-counter supplements, which often contain just one herb and, because of a pretty unregulated market, may even contain poor-quality ingredients.' She stresses that a nuanced understanding of how herbs interact with the body and with each other is essential, and that 'hit-and-miss' purchasing of single over-the-counter remedies may therefore fail to deliver the desired results.

'Herbal medicine can be a safe, effective and important part of your menopause and recovery toolkit. Do your research, buy quality products, get expert advice if needed and start with taking one herbal medicine at a time so you can get a clear idea of how it feels for you,' is her advice.

Everyone is different – what works for one person may not work for you.

Vitamins, Minerals and Other Supplements

Questions about supplements come up almost daily in our Facebook community. People ask for recommendations and share what they take. Some are looking for a supplement to help ease a menopause symptom, some want to support their health in general, while others are concerned about whether certain supplements are safe for them. All are valid points to consider and, with over 90,000 supplements out there on the market, it is undoubtedly a confusing area to navigate.

Some healthcare professionals claim that supplements don't work – full stop. They argue that if you maintain a balanced diet, you can obtain all the necessary nutrients from food alone, making supplementation unnecessary. While this approach works in theory, it may not reflect the reality for everyone. Factors like modern farming practices, nutrient depletion in soil, busy lifestyles and individual health conditions can make it difficult to get all the essential nutrients from diet alone.

I've met many cancer survivors who struggle to maintain a varied and balanced diet for extended periods of time. Side effects of treatment, such as loss of appetite, nausea, mouth ulcers and more, often make eating a healthy diet an unrealistic expectation during these challenging times. That's where others, myself included, believe supplements can play an important role, filling gaps in nutrition and supporting overall health. Additionally, I have spoken to many doctors who believe that specific supplements can help to ease symptoms. It's about finding balance and understanding that, while food should be the primary source of nutrients, supplements can be a helpful addition when needed. (See also pages 165–176, where I discuss herbal supplements in detail.)

It's also very important to note that supplement markets lack regulation, and that vitamin and mineral supplements should never be a substitute for a healthy diet. And more is not always better; too high a dose of certain vitamins and minerals can have adverse effects. Therefore, it's crucial to stick to the daily recommended dose or the dose as recommended by your healthcare practitioner to ensure safety and effectiveness. Personally, since my cancer diagnosis, my approach to food has evolved. I became vegan overnight without much knowledge about nutrition, then reintroduced fish into my diet a few years later. Looking back, I realise there were times when I probably wasn't getting all the nutrients I needed from my diet alone. At the time, I didn't know any better, so I didn't consider taking supplements to fill the gaps, such as vitamin B or omega-3s. And I know my dietary intake of calcium was low, because I tracked it. But I've learned, and I want to pass on what I've discovered, not just because it might help with your menopause symptoms but to help you take a holistic approach to self-care.

The supplements I've chosen to consider in this section are those that are discussed most frequently in conversations with our community.

Before we dive in, however, I think you need to start by asking yourself why you want to take a dietary supplement.

1. Is it to help manage a specific symptom?

2. Is it a 'just in case I don't get enough from food' type scenario?

3. Or perhaps you feel you want to support your future health the best way you can?

The clearer you can be about your why, the more straightforward will be your research into what you may benefit from. You also really want to avoid being in the situation of having a cupboard full of supplements and not quite knowing what they are each for; or worse, taking supplements that have adverse effects or bad interactions. There were times in my recovery when I had drawers full of bottles, pills and powders and in total honesty I had no real plan about what they were and why I was taking all of them. But in my quest to heal, it seemed like a good idea at the time! So I am hoping that, instead of doing what I did (and wasting quite a lot of money), this section is going to help you be a little more structured in your approach. Understanding how these supplements work and the situations in which they are most effective can be incredibly valuable when deciding your next steps. For instance, I provide tips on calculating your daily calcium intake, which can be both eye-opening and empowering, helping you make informed decisions about what actions to take moving forward.

Whenever I speak to an integrative medical doctor they will tell me that the best way to work with supplements is to know whether you are deficient, or to have undergone tests to help you understand what's going on in your body, instead of just guessing. And of course that makes sense, but we also know that not everyone has access to doctors who can help you do that. There are, however, some things you can test for that may be helpful for you in determining whether you need a dietary supplement or not.

Before you even go down the complicated supplement route, consider getting some basic blood tests done – your vitamin D and vitamin B levels and your ferritin levels, for example. Some of the menopause symptoms you are experiencing could be attributable to other conditions and not just a lack of hormones. In one of our workshops, when a participant asked what she could do about her restless legs, one of our menopause specialist doctors suggested that she start by checking her ferritin levels with a basic blood test, as restless legs can be caused by low levels of ferritin. In the UK, you can ask your GP to have these levels checked for you.

Multivitamins

Multivitamins can help fill nutritional gaps in the diet, providing essential vitamins and minerals that support overall health and immunity. If you're in the 'just in case I don't get enough nutrients from food' group and are considering a multivitamin for that reason, make sure to read the ingredients list. You may be better to take a standard multivitamin, rather than one aimed at perimenopausal and menopausal women, because many menopause multivitamin supplements contain ingredients that may have potential contraindications for you. For instance, some multivitamin supplements may contain phytoestrogens, and, as we discuss in the herbal medicine section, in concentrated form they are not advised for women with a history of hormone-sensitive cancers. Other multivitamins might contain ingredients such as turmeric; if you're on tamoxifen, for example, turmeric in concentrated form is contraindicated because it may interfere with the drug's effectiveness (for more information, see pages 187–188).

In researching for this book, I came across some findings from randomised trials of multivitamins that reveal a significant effect on memory in older adults.[75] Since I know that cognitive decline is a major worry for many of our community, especially those who are in early menopause after cancer, I wanted to add this here. 'It's unlikely that a single nutrient is a magic bullet and dietary supplements will never be a substitute for a healthy diet,' explains Professor JoAnn Manson, a prominent researcher and physician known for her work in preventive medicine and women's health.

She continues, 'Several micronutrients are known to be important for optimal brain health, and a deficiency of one or more of those essential vitamins and minerals could accelerate cognitive ageing. The finding that a daily multivitamin improved memory and slowed cognitive ageing in three separate placebo-controlled studies in COSMOS is exciting and further supports the promise of multivitamins as a safe, accessible and affordable approach to protecting cognitive health in older adults.'[76]

Vitamin D

Vitamin D is important for healthy bones because it helps you absorb calcium from your diet, which again is important for your bone health. Additionally, it plays an important role in the function of our immune system. In 2016, the UK's Department of Health updated its guidelines to acknowledge that many people in the UK struggle to maintain adequate vitamin D levels for optimal health. The primary source of vitamin D is sunlight, but achieving sufficient levels can be particularly challenging during the winter months and due to the widespread use of sunscreen throughout the year. And while certain foods, like trout, salmon, tuna and mushrooms, as well as fortified products like cereals, also offer some vitamin D, it is unlikely that people in the UK are obtaining enough from diet and sunlight alone.[77] Government recommendations in the UK and in many parts of the world state that from October to March everyone should consider taking a daily supplement containing 10 micrograms (400 IU – International Units) of vitamin D daily. If your blood levels show deficient levels of vitamin D, then you may need to add a supplement.

I know that most of you reading this have already been diagnosed with cancer, but it's interesting to note that several studies show that vitamin D deficiency has been linked to several types of cancer, including prostate, multiple myeloma, colorectal and breast cancer.[78] Some studies suggest that higher levels of vitamin D may lower the risk of cancer-related deaths, while others propose that it could be a potential risk factor. So, get your vitamin D levels checked – and make sure that you are in the optimum range; remember, more is not better. The British Heart Foundations says, 'Don't take very high doses of vitamin D, as if you do this over a long period of time, it can cause too much calcium to build up in the body, which can weaken the bones and damage the kidneys and heart.'

You can choose from pills, sprays, capsules, gummies and drops. At home, we call our vitamin D supplements 'sunshine in a bottle', and it feels empowering to me knowing how much it supports my overall health.

Calcium

The mineral calcium is well known to be important for strong bones and teeth, and also for healthy muscle and nerve function. Unlike vitamin D, however, it is very possible that you get enough calcium from your diet and may not need a supplement. Some women do get a calcium supplement prescribed by their doctor, but unless this is the case for you it is not advised to take calcium supplements, as too much may increase your risk of other health problems.

The Royal Osteoporosis Society advises that adults in the UK need to consume 700mg of calcium a day, or 1000mg if you are on osteoporosis medication or have osteoporosis.[79] But of course it's hard to know what that could look like in your diet or if you are getting enough. Do you have any idea?

The International Osteoporosis Foundation has a really good and easy-to-use calculator on their website that helps you work out how much calcium on average you consume a week. I've linked the webpage in your digital handbook for you. You just tick off what you eat and it is a really helpful exercise that I'd recommend you do. When I did mine, my calculated calcium intake was too low; I came in at 600mg and it is recommended for me to have 1000mg a day as I have a diagnosis of osteopenia. This was really surprising for me as I feel I have a good diet containing plenty of whole foods. But it also meant I could do something about it. For example, I started to add three apricots to my breakfast oats, and that alone increased my intake by 120mg a day. I also stopped using organic soya milk for my tea and coffee and switched to nonorganic versions, as these are fortified and include about the same amount of calcium as dairy milk. By focusing on adding more calcium-rich foods to my week's food and making some swaps, I was able to meet the recommended amounts. I feel much better knowing that I can achieve my recommended calcium intake by making small tweaks.

So, please do get tracking your calcium intake. It is empowering and a good exercise to do for sure.

You can find calcium in dairy products, tofu and other soya-based foods, leafy green veg, fortified plant milks, sardines, chickpeas, edamame beans and other beans and lentils, as well as nuts and seeds and some dried fruit. A calcium supplement is only helpful when prescribed by your doctor specifically for you.

Vitamin B

Vitamin B plays a crucial role in energy production, brain function and mood regulation, helping to reduce fatigue, stress and cognitive decline, particularly during menopause. Despite this, vitamin B doesn't always get the attention it deserves, which is why I wanted to focus on it here. After a cancer diagnosis, many people focus on improving their diet by adding more fruits and vegetables, and some, like myself, may adopt a plant-focused lifestyle. However, while other B vitamins are abundant in plant-based foods, vitamin B12 is not (it's mainly found in animal products like meat, fish, eggs and dairy), so if you're vegan or vegetarian it's important to ensure you're getting enough. Vegans often need to rely on fortified foods or supplements for this. If you're low in B12, you may feel more tired, adding to your menopause symptoms, so it's important to monitor your levels.

Magnesium

Magnesium is essential for many bodily functions, including supporting muscle and nerve function, regulating blood pressure and promoting healthy bones. It can also aid in reducing muscle cramps and improving sleep.[80] Magnesium is an important mineral for brain function too.

Studies suggest that magnesium supplements may help with a number of menopause symptoms, including anxiety, low mood and reduced bone density, and in our Facebook community this is the most frequently discussed supplement. Many women claim that taking magnesium before bedtime helps them sleep better. British Menopause Society recognised expert, founder of Myla Health, a menopause clinic, and sleep specialist Dr Zoe Schaedel, however, says, 'There is little evidence that magnesium aids sleep, and it does not feature in any of the sleep guidelines. But I've spoken to lots of women who say that it helps their sleep.' So, if you feel it helps you, then it's worth pursuing.

Many women enquire about what type of magnesium to take because once you start exploring it can be confusing knowing which one to opt for. Magnesium is available in various forms, including pills, tablets, creams and sprays, as well as a wide variety of formulations and strengths. For menopausal symptoms, magnesium glycinate is the one you're most likely to need, but I've also given you an explanation of some of the other most common forms. Integrative medicine expert Dr Shelly Latte-Naor of the Memorial Sloan Kettering Cancer Center in New York adds, 'Magnesium can have a laxative effect for some people – especially magnesium oxide and citrate. This may or may not be preferential.'

Magnesium glycinate: This form is the most popular due to its calming effects – it is also used in bath salts for muscle relaxation and soreness relief.

Magnesium sulfate: Commonly known as Epsom salts, it's often used in baths for muscle relaxation and relief of soreness.

Magnesium citrate: Often used to support digestion and relieve constipation.

Magnesium oxide: A common and inexpensive form, often used to relieve digestive issues.

Collagen

Collagen is a protein that is particularly important for skin because it provides structure, elasticity and hydration. It supports the strength and flexibility of connective tissues, helping to maintain bone density and reduce joint pain or stiffness by improving cartilage health. Given that so many people in our community say things like, 'I feel like an old lady since my cancer treatment-induced menopause,' and 'My joint ache is so bad,' or 'My skin is as dry as a prune,' it is understandable that one might feel that a collagen supplement is a good supplement to invest in.

As I am writing this book there is a lot of hype around collagen, and I think some people feel they are missing out if they are not taking it. While researching for an episode on the subject for The Menopause and Cancer Podcast, I was exploring social media to see which brands are available. Within an hour, I noticed that my Instagram algorithm was bombarding me with brands showing me their products, and I was confused right from the start. Is liquid collagen best, or powder? Derived from animal sources, such as bovine (cow), porcine (pig) or marine (fish), or a vegan option? With or without added vitamins? Gosh, it was confusing.

But there was one question that worried me more than anything. I had heard somewhere that collagen supplements may promote cancer cell growth. And in the past, just hearing that had meant I had stayed away from it altogether.

So when I asked integrative oncologist Dr Nina Fuller-Shavel if people with a history of cancer can safely take collagen to aid our menopausal symptoms, she told me: 'The question is very difficult because we actually don't have enough evidence at the moment. There's a misconception about collagen supplements being linked to tumour growth due to confusion surrounding the collagen present in tumours. However, the collagen we consume orally as supplements is unrelated to tumour collagen. There's no evidence of a direct negative link between oral collagen and tumour growth. However, there's a lack of robust studies on collagen's safety and effectiveness in individuals with a history of cancer. Existing research mainly focuses on generally healthy individuals or those with specific health issues, like joint problems or skin elasticity loss, rather than cancer survivors or those undergoing treatment.'

For those considering a collagen supplement, Dr Fuller-Shavel recommends opting for a pure collagen powder with minimal added ingredients. She explains, 'Liquid collagen products often contain additives such as stabilisers, sweeteners and preservatives, which are best avoided when choosing a supplement. Choosing a pure powder allows for easier ingredient checking and ensures that only necessary components are consumed, avoiding unnecessary additives that may not be beneficial to health.' Dr Fuller-Shavel suggests that if you're considering trying any new intervention, such as a supplement, it's important to ask your pharmacist or doctor to confirm that there are no interactions with any of the medication you are on. And if you don't notice any benefits within six to eight weeks of use, it may not be the right intervention for you and you should consider trying something else or seeking further support.

Turmeric

> *'Hi all, I've been taking turmeric supplements for joint pain but just read we shouldn't be as it might interfere with tamoxifen. Any truth in this?'*

We get a lot of questions like this in our Facebook group. People also often ask if turmeric and curcumin are the same, and the answer is no, but they are related.[81] Turmeric is a bright yellow spice that is native to South-east Asia. Curcumin is a bioactive compound, the major one in turmeric, that gives it its distinctive colour. Curcumin has been shown to have several valuable properties including being anti-inflammatory, metabolic-regulating, immune-modulating and mood-enhancing, and it even has anti-cancer benefits.[82]

Many menopause-blend supplements contain concentrated doses of curcumin. When I asked Rebekah Brown, founder of menopause supplement brand Mpowder, to explain to me what our community needs to be aware of, she advised: 'Using turmeric as a spice in cooking is considered safe after cancer, when incorporated into a balanced diet. Cooking with turmeric adds flavour to dishes without necessarily providing high concentrations of curcumin. Remember that curcumin is usually poorly absorbed, and that the addition of black pepper and fat to a dish increases its bioavailability.

Mpowder's website contains further information about taking turmeric and curcumin with a history of cancer.[83]

Dr Latte-Naor says, 'There is also a theory that the high antioxidant potential of curcumin may counter the effect of some chemotherapy agents or radiation. Additionally, higher amounts can have a blood-thinning effect, which is why we advise patients to stop their high-dose turmeric/curcumin prior to surgery. At this stage, if undergoing active cancer treatment for breast cancer it is advisable to check with your healthcare provider before taking turmeric in the form of a supplement.'

Psychological Therapies

Psychological therapies, such as CBT, CBT-I, talking therapy, counselling, hypnotherapy and other strategies, can provide valuable support for managing emotional and mental challenges for cancer survivors. These approaches help address issues like stress, anxiety, low mood and sleep problems among others, offering practical tools for improving overall wellbeing.

CBT, CBT-I, talking therapy, counselling and hypnotherapy

Coping with, understanding and accepting your cancer diagnosis and the uncertainty it brings with it can have a huge impact on your mental health. Feelings like anger, not feeling like yourself any more, having lost your mojo and motivation, feelings of low mood (if this persists we talk about depression), irritability, anxiety, low self-esteem and loss of confidence are all symptoms you may be experiencing. And often, it can be impossible to know exactly what is going on and why you are feeling the way you do.

Depression can manifest as physical pain through a variety of symptoms, including aches and pains, insomnia, digestive issues or headaches. Physical pain, on the other hand, can lead to feelings of low mood and depression. Menopause and low oestrogen levels can also affect your mood and emotions.

In the months and early years after my active cancer treatment finished, when I no longer had any cancer present in my body and my doctors had given me the good news that I was in remission, my mental health was at an all-time low. I received some counselling sessions from my hospital; however, I never really felt I 'clicked' with my counsellor. She didn't say much and, although I understand that there are different approaches, I think at that point I needed a little more conversation. After the hospital sessions came to an end, I went on to find a therapist privately. I was struggling a lot and knew I needed help. Besides, my mum is a therapist and always encouraged me to pursue this as support. I am so glad I listened to her. The therapist I found worked with a whole range of therapeutic models. She explained that, while we would base our work together on traditional talking therapy, she might also use strategies like CBT (cognitive behavioural therapy), as well as mind–body based approaches like EFT (emotional freedom technique), which is an alternative treatment for physical pain and emotional distress. At that point I had felt so distressed on a daily basis that I was willing to try anything. For the first few sessions all I did was cry. I felt exhausted afterwards, but in a good way. My sessions with my therapist became the time in my week where I could let it all spill out ,and that felt good.

Through therapy I began to realise that many of my thoughts were spiralling into worst-case scenarios almost all the time. Any little ache in my body would lead me to think, 'Is this the cancer back?' I'd then doubt myself, thinking, 'No, don't be silly, Dani, you've just pulled a muscle in yoga.' But the anxiety would continue: 'Should I phone the breast care nurse?' I'd then decide, 'No, now's not a good time, I'll do it after the holidays.' The cycle of worry was relentless: 'If I do ring the doctors, will they recommend a scan? How will I cope with scanxiety? What if this is cancer? How will I tell the girls that Mummy's cancer is back?'

This spiralling anxiety had me in its grip and I could not escape it. My thoughts, it seemed, were always quicker than me. They came in uninvited and were always there, from the moment I opened my eyes in the morning until I went to bed at night. A lot of that anxiety was irrational, of course. In my mind I saw my oncologist tell me that my cancer was back endless times. I remember a couple of occasions when it all felt too much and I wondered how big the relief would be if it all stopped, if life stopped. Isn't it crazy to think that in a time where I was so desperately trying to survive, the end of life would seem like a relief? It makes no sense when viewed rationally, but depression and anxiety aren't rational. Today, I know I was depressed.

I did not share my worries with many people, but sometimes well-meaning and loving people would suggest just keeping busy and distracting myself. But for me, that never really worked. Even while juggling the demands of three young kids, each scooting off in a different direction for school, my mind somehow managed to keep those fear-of-recurrence conversations going in a loop in my head. At first I couldn't trust my body, and now I couldn't trust my mind either. I felt so out of control. My quality of life was deeply impacted by my psychological state and, no matter how much I tried to push those thoughts away, they were always there.

Physically, however, I was doing so much better. I completed a half marathon in exactly two hours, only nine months after my active cancer treatment finished; but my mental health was in slow-motion recovery.

CBT for menopause symptoms

One day, my therapist got a pen and paper out and helped me look at my repetitive cycle of thoughts. We named my fears and instead of pushing them away we allowed them all to be there, visible on paper. It became apparent that my thoughts affected how I felt physically (I suffered anxiety symptoms, like racing heart and panic attacks) and also emotionally (I was scared and exhausted), and this was having an impact on my actions (I couldn't make decisions, even about when to call the breast care nurse or plan for the future). I didn't know it then, but we were using the model of CBT (cognitive behavioural therapy) to help me through this tough time.

CBT aims to stop negative cycles by changing your negative thought patterns – breaking down things that make you feel bad, anxious or scared. By making your problems more manageable, CBT can improve the way you feel. It is such a powerful model, with plenty of evidence to back up its effectiveness.

The Women's Health Concern factsheet on cognitive behavioural therapy for menopausal symptoms states that: CBT is a brief, non-medical approach that can be helpful for a range of health problems, including anxiety and stress, depressed mood, hot flushes and night sweats, sleep problems and fatigue. CBT helps people to develop practical ways of managing problems and provides new coping skills and useful strategies. For this reason, it can be a helpful approach to try because the skills can be applied to different problems, and can improve wellbeing in general.[84]

Professor Myra Hunter, from King's College London, is an expert in cognitive behavioural therapy (CBT) and how it can be used to help women during the menopause. Her book *Managing Hot Flushes and Night Sweats: A Cognitive Behavioural Self-Help Guide to the Menopause* is very helpful.

CBT for anxiety

Here's an example of how CBT provided help for my anxiety around recurrence:

> **Problem:** *I am constantly worried that my cancer might return. These thoughts often interfere with daily life, causing significant anxiety and distress.*
>
> **Step 1: Identify negative thoughts**
>
> *I realised that I frequently think, 'Any small pain or change in my body means my cancer is back.'*
>
> **Step 2: Challenge negative thoughts**
>
> *My CBT therapist helped me question these thoughts by asking, 'What evidence do you have that every pain means cancer recurrence?' and, 'Have you experienced these symptoms before without it being cancer?' I acknowledged that I have had various aches and pains that were not related to cancer in the past (it's called being human!).*
>
> **Step 3: Reframe thoughts**
>
> *Together, we worked on reframing my thoughts. Instead of thinking, 'This pain means my cancer is back,' I learned to think, 'I have experienced similar symptoms before, and they were not related to cancer. I will monitor them and consult my doctor if they persist.' My oncologist helped at one stage and suggested I make notes in my diary when I experienced symptoms and*

then put another date in my diary for six weeks' time to check in with myself and to review my situation. She suggested that this might help me not obsess over my symptoms every single day, wondering what to do with them. If my symptoms persisted, I would contact them. This allowed me to 'park' my constant thinking about when to call – whether to call – and gave me a roadmap, helping me focus on managing my symptoms without the added stress of indecision.

Step 4: Behaviour strategies

I also learned that relaxation techniques such as mindfulness and progressive muscle relaxation help manage anxiety. I had learned these tools in yoga, but strangely it had not occurred to me to use them off the yoga mat too.

Outcome:

By identifying, challenging and reframing my negative thoughts, and employing relaxation techniques, I found that my anxiety about cancer recurrence decreased over time. I felt a little more in control of my thoughts and emotions, which enabled me to enjoy my daily life more fully.

If you have worries or anxieties, of any type or severity, please know you're not alone, and reach out to others and experts who can help you. And if you need to talk to someone now, the Samaritans have a 24-hour phone line.

CBT for physical symptoms

Can CBT work in addressing a physical symptom? There has recently been media attention on CBT being a helpful tool for managing hot flushes. This led to controversy; some people said it was suggesting that our symptoms are all in our heads. Of course, it's not that simple!

Several randomised control trials indicate that CBT can be effective for hot flushes. Hot flushes and night sweats are experienced by up to 85 per cent of people after breast cancer, and they can have a significant impact on sleep and quality of life, as well as having consequences for employment and personal relationships.[85] Given the data on how many people struggle with them, I want to go into detail here to ensure we all know how it works. CBT is *not* going to reduce the severity of your hot flushes, but it can help with how they impact you – and that is where the benefit lies.

- CBT helps individuals become aware of the negative thoughts that arise before and during hot flushes. These thoughts often include worries and catastrophic thinking such as, 'If I get a hot flush now, it'll be so embarrassing', or, 'This is unbearable', or 'Everyone can see I'm sweating'.

- Through CBT, you can learn to challenge these negative thoughts and reframe them into more positive, neutral and realistic ones. For example, replacing 'This is unbearable' with, 'This is uncomfortable, but I can manage it' or, 'I've dealt with hot flushes before and I know they will pass'.

- CBT incorporates relaxation techniques such as deep breathing, progressive muscle relaxation and mindfulness meditation to help manage the physical symptoms of hot flushes. It can make a big difference to how you experience the hot flush if you teach yourself to take some deep and conscious breaths, rather than frantically reacting to the discomfort; this will allow you to maintain a sense of calm and regain control in those moments.

- Since stress can also trigger or worsen hot flushes, CBT focuses on teaching stress management skills. This can include time management, setting realistic goals and practising self-care. Working on our overall stress levels can have an impact on physical symptoms.

- CBT helps build resilience by encouraging positive coping strategies and a proactive approach to managing symptoms.

CBT-I (Cognitive Behavioural Therapy for Insomnia)

If you struggle to fall asleep when you go to bed, or wake up in the middle of the night and can't go back to sleep, and this happens at least three times a week for more than three months, it can usually be diagnosed as chronic insomnia,' says Dr Zoe Schaedel. As well as being a menopause specialist and running a busy NHS clinic, Dr Schaedel is the founder of the Good Sleep Clinic; few people are as expertly equipped to advise cancer survivors in menopause with sleep problems.

'There are lots of studies showing if you use cognitive behavioural therapy for insomnia, in 70–80 per cent of cases sufferers can recover from that insomnia. Even if you're on medication like tamoxifen or letrozole, CBT-I can help. It can help you cope with those awakenings and make them less disruptive, allowing you to get back to sleep quicker,' she says.

Research reveals that in cancer patients or survivors, CBT-I is associated with statistically and clinically significant improvements in sleep outcomes. CBT-I may also improve mood, fatigue and overall quality of life.[86]

Dr Schaedel goes on to elaborate that CBT-I is a specific programme that also educates people about what happens with our brains in the middle of the night. 'At night, things can feel much worse. Your brain works differently then; it's driven by the amygdala, the part of the brain that feels anxiety. The prefrontal cortex, which provides logical functioning, doesn't activate properly at night as it does during the day,' she says. This was such a good explanation for me as it's so true: all my thoughts are so much worse at night! During the times when I was highly anxious and I couldn't sleep very well, I'd sometimes get into my kids' beds and sleep with them as a means of distracting myself. Luckily they enjoyed my midnight snuggles!

What's so good about CBT-I is that it can help reset your sleep patterns and can be effective long-term. A programme usually lasts about six weeks and focuses on relearning and rewiring your behaviour.

What's important to remember is that embarking on a course of CBT-I is a project. It will require some of your thinking space; and it's a practice, so it will also require some level of effort. In some cases the programme has you getting out of bed in the night (I know! This sounds so counterintuitive when all you want to do is sleep) to re-teach your brain and body that the bedroom is for sleeping.

Here, Dr Schaedel shares a practical example of how CBT-I can work; but remember that it will look slightly different for each person.

> *Sarah has started to experience insomnia after starting tamoxifen for her breast cancer treatment. She frequently wakes*

up in the middle of the night and struggles to fall back asleep. Sarah knows how important sleep is and has been getting really anxious about her sleep. Even before she goes to bed she will worry about what it's going to be like.

Sarah is advised by her clinician to keep a sleep diary, noting her sleep patterns and any night-time waking. She notices a pattern of waking up around 2am and struggling to fall back to sleep for hours. Just as she drifts off, her alarm goes off and she has to wake her children for school. She can feel her adrenaline pump through her. 'I just feel dreadful all day,' she says. It is normal to have disturbed sleep from time to time, particularly in someone who has stress or worry associated with a cancer diagnosis. Usually this type of sleep disruption settles quite quickly but, if sleep continues to be disturbed for some time, a kind of habit often develops where the body and brain get used to lying awake for hours at night. This can itself become part of the problem, and an important part of CBT-I is trying to reduce the amount of the night that you are lying awake in bed.

Sarah and her clinician use Sarah's sleep diary to work on sleep restriction and stimulus control; her clinician finds that she is spending about ten hours in bed at night, but is only asleep for five hours. This is called 'poor sleep efficiency'. Sarah is advised to limit her time in bed to five and a half hours, from midnight to 5.30am. She is also advised only to go to bed when she feels very sleepy and to get out of bed if she can't sleep after 20 minutes. Very quickly Sarah starts to have longer bursts of more continuous, better-quality sleep. Her clinician advises her that she can gradually increase the time she remains in bed each week.

Sarah also starts working on changing her thoughts about sleep, a technique called cognitive restructuring. Instead of worrying about not sleeping, she practises telling herself that waking up is manageable and she will be able to cope even if she does not get a full night's sleep. She also reminds herself that humankind has often managed to go without sleep for prolonged periods of time and that she will be okay.

Sarah has also learned new relaxation techniques for her bedtime routine. She practises deep breathing exercises and progressive muscle relaxation to reduce anxiety and physical tension before bed. She finds that plugging herself into audio recordings works best for her.

Continued practice: 'Sarah continues with these techniques; continued practice is very important. She adjusts her sleep window as her sleep efficiency improves. She starts spending more time in bed as her sleep becomes more consolidated.

Over the six-week period, Sarah notices a significant improvement in her sleep. She feels her waking is becoming less disruptive and she finds it easier to fall back asleep. The anxiety about her sleep diminishes and she feels more rested and better able to manage her daily activities. Sarah still has some nights where she wakes up at 2am, but she is much less worried about that now that she has a plan for what to do.

I hope this explanation helps show you how important it is to invest time and effort into CBT-I.

What I love most about Dr Schaedel's approach is her practical and empathetic desire to help as many people as possible. She adds that, although it is easier with direct support, books can be really helpful, and recommends in particular *How to Beat Insomnia and Sleep Problems One Step at a Time* by Kirstie Anderson.

So whether you've decided to dive into a book, follow an online programme or take a one-on-one course, I hope you now have a better understanding of how CBT-I can help. Remember, it does require some effort and commitment, and it's perfectly okay if you're not ready for that right now. Just know that it's a strategy you can revisit whenever you feel prepared to take it on.

As a final note, sometimes addressing other symptoms before focusing on your sleep can be helpful; for example, if you wake up due to severe night sweats, it may be more effective to manage those symptoms first before tackling CBT-I. Turn to pages 304–308 to get an overview of all you can do to help address your sleep-related symptoms.

CBT and CBT-I are more than just a treatment; they're almost a 'learning for life' approach that offers benefits beyond what you might initially expect. Through CBT and CBT-I you gain valuable insights into yourself, which is incredibly beneficial. However, I understand that fitting it into a busy schedule, especially when juggling children, a job and other commitments, can be challenging. If it feels overwhelming right now, that's perfectly understandable.

How to access CBT and CBT-I

It's important to add that access to CBT and CBT-I isn't always straightforward. It can vary depending on your location, healthcare system and the resources available. CBT and CBT-I can be done in a one-on-one setting, as in my case for example, or in a group setting or through structured online learning.

- Many people start by discussing their symptoms with their primary care doctor, who can provide a referral to a therapist or a mental health specialist.
- In the UK, CBT is available through the NHS. You can also self-refer through the NHS Talking Therapies for Anxiety and Depression Programme.[87]
- You can search for licensed CBT practitioners privately and contact them directly for appointments. This may involve out-of-pocket costs if not covered by insurance.
- It might also be worth it to try to contact a few of your local cancer charities to see if they run some sessions, as many do.
- There are also various online programmes and apps that offer CBT-based resources and guided self-help modules.
- For CBT-I specifically, Dr Schaedel points out that there are some excellent online programmes, such as Sleepio, Sleepstation and Sleepful, which can guide you through the CBT-I model step by step. Depending on your location, these programmes might be available for free or through your GP; for instance, in the UK the charity Macmillan has partnered with Sleepio.

Talking therapy and counselling

In all my many years of working with people affected by cancer, I've not met anyone who didn't suffer from a decline in their mental health – for a period of time, at least. Getting a cancer diagnosis is a huge shock, and starting treatment can feel terrifying, especially when you don't know exactly what to expect. And then there's the worry of all the what ifs; facing our own mortality can bring up so much fear.

As most of us have experienced, even after active treatment it can be a struggle to move forward and embrace our 'new normal'. That's where counselling and therapy can come in. Of course, they're not a direct treatment for menopause symptoms, but I couldn't write this chapter without acknowledging just how valuable they can be for us survivors. To share distressing thoughts or your biggest fears or anxieties with a professional who you trust can be hugely helpful. Counselling and therapy can complement approaches such as CBT, CBT-I and various other strategies, offering additional support for emotional and mental wellbeing.

Counselling typically focuses on providing guidance, support and practical solutions to help individuals address specific problems, improve coping skills and achieve specific goals. Counselling sessions may be short-term and focused on addressing immediate concerns. Therapy, on the other hand, is a broader term that encompasses a range of therapeutic approaches aimed at addressing underlying psychological issues. Therapy sessions may be longer-term and delve deeper into exploring emotions, thoughts, beliefs and past experiences that contribute to mental health concerns. Many therapists use different approaches, methods or techniques to treat patients or address specific conditions, including CBT, psychodynamic therapy, acceptance and commitment therapy, and mindfulness-based approaches.

Just after I had finished my active cancer treatment, my husband Tim sought the help of a counsellor from a Macmillan centre at one of our local hospitals, where they offer support to family members of those affected by cancer. Cancer is, after all, a family affair and hugely impacts those around us as well. It's a lot to cope with for everyone. He explains what led him to seek that help.

> *'It was about eight months in and there were lots of telltale signs that I was finding it hard to cope. I'd left my watch in a cubicle at the gym, I blew up the battery on the car, had a car accident... There was one day when I was in a card shop, and the lady behind the counter said, "Are you okay?" And I said, "I don't think I am." I must have stood there for about 40 minutes, just staring into space. So I went and asked for counselling and it was hugely helpful. It's so easy to go down a dark hole but the counsellor helped me think of where we were at that point, to keep focusing on the now, which kept me present and helped me worry less about the future. That was really key. I would say to anyone going through it, of course you're going to go down a path of asking, what happens if this happens and that happens. But if you look at where you are now, that can be very helpful.'*

I can't stress enough how important it is to take a moment for yourself and think about whether you could benefit from counselling or therapy. Consider speaking to your GP or your cancer team, who will hopefully be able to refer you. Contact your local charities too, as they might offer support. You may be wondering, 'Am I bad enough to seek help?' I hear this all the time – that women believe they have to feel really bad and at rock bottom before they can go and seek help. But I'd like to question that. Therapy or counselling can be such helpful additions to your post-survivorship toolkit. You have much to process, and it takes a lot to come to grips with the fact that you are now menopausal as well. Talking about it in a safe space can be transformative.

The Benefits of Community

Since we are delving into the options of emotional and mental health support, I must bring up the benefit of community. I have seen, over and over again, how beneficial it can be to connect to others in a similar situation. In the UK, the charity Breast Cancer Now offers moving-forward courses, and the peer-to-peer support is hugely helpful for improving mental health. Some people might find an online cancer survivor group more suited to them. You're also welcome to join our private Facebook group, the Menopause and Cancer Chat Hub, where you can pop in, ask questions or simply sit back and read. Hearing and reading others' stories can make you feel less alone.

Hypnotherapy

Hypnotherapy is a type of therapy where a trained therapist uses guided hypnosis to help individuals achieve a state of focused attention and heightened suggestibility. When you are in this relaxed state, the therapist can help you explore thoughts, feelings and memories. People can come with any issue, such as anxiety, stress, phobias, pain management or behavioural changes. The aim is to facilitate positive change by accessing the subconscious mind, allowing you to reframe negative patterns and reinforce healthier behaviours.

I spoke to hypnotherapist Debbie Pugh, who works at the Cambridge Cancer Help Centre and has helped cancer patients better manage their problems with hypnotherapy for decades. Debbie explains, 'People can come with any problem. I'd like to stress that hypnosis is a complementary therapy to something like counselling. So in hypnotherapy, yes, we're having conversations with the person regarding the presenting problems. So if they're feeling stressed and anxious, then that's what we will work with them on. But if they have something like trauma or other presenting challenges, I might refer them to someone who is a specialist in that area to support them.'

After having spoken to Debbie, I was curious about how exactly hypnotherapy can help cancer patients – and, more precisely, help manage menopausal symptoms. I asked Dr Shelly Latte-Naor of the Memorial Sloan Kettering Cancer Center in New York, who has special training in therapies and treatments that go along with cancer care, about hypnotherapy.

'Research suggests that self-hypnosis has the potential to help women with a history of cancer and it can help reduce or manage the effects of symptoms such as pain and fatigue. There is also evidence that hypnotic treatment may reduce the frequency and severity of hot flushes and may also improve sleep quality in breast cancer survivors, both as we know issues that affect a large proportion of survivors,' Dr Latte-Naor explained.

She adds that, during hypnotherapy, you enter a relaxed state of being and you can also work with using visual imagery. You can imagine placing your face in a freezer, feeling the refreshing cold spread to your neck and chest, or your feet in a bucket of iced water. By practising these imagery techniques, you can learn to bring them to mind for relief – for example, when you feel you are coming on with a hot flush while sitting in a meeting you can picture the iced water.

Similarly to CBT, hypnotherapy can be done in a one-to-one setting or a group setting. Also similarly, in many cases accessing it might be an issue. In the UK, I have heard from several patients who have joined online group hypnotherapy courses that they were able to access through charities. The support is out there, and I encourage you to search for sources of access to it should you wish to explore this further.

Yoga

I first stepped onto the yoga mat because my mother-in-law had suggested I go to a local class in a village hall. My first few classes were consumed by my worrying about my wig slipping off my head in downward dog. In fact it was a slippery affair all round, as I had lost my big toenails during chemotherapy, so I was too embarrassed to show my feet and kept my socks on. But gradually, I began to feel a sense of calm and trust. Yoga became a vehicle of hope for me. It felt like I was slowly rebuilding my battered physical body and healing emotionally by grounding myself in the present. During the hours on the mat, I felt less anxious about the 'what ifs', more anchored in the present moment. It was bliss. Relief. So much so that I decided to become a yoga teacher, so that I could share this powerful technique with others too.

Having taught hundreds of students over the years, I understand what might stop you from stepping on the mat. Many people say they are not flexible enough to do yoga, that they can't touch their toes or they could not sit and meditate. But that's exactly why you go to yoga: to improve your flexibility and strength over time. Yoga is for everyone, and it's as much about giving your mind a break as strengthening or stretching out your body. Think of it as an MOT for your mind. It's about listening to your body, setting achievable goals and celebrating small improvements, rather than striving for perfection.

Yoga's benefits go beyond physical exercise. Rooted in ancient Indian tradition, it combines meditation, breathing techniques and movement to nurture the body, mind and spirit. Research suggests that it can have a profound impact on cancer survivors. Over thirty-four randomised control trials have shown that yoga improves physical function, mental health and quality of life of cancer survivors.[88] There is also plenty of research showing that yoga significantly reduces cancer-related fatigue and improves physical activity and sleep quality.[89] Furthermore, a 2023 study presented at the ASCO (American Society of Clinical Oncology) annual meeting found that yoga reduced inflammation among cancer survivors, as reported in the *Guardian* in 2023.[90] This randomised control trial demonstrated that yoga participants had significantly lower levels of pro-inflammatory markers compared to those attending health education classes.

To me, all of the above means that yoga is well worth investigating if you are living with menopause symptoms after cancer. Yoga is easily accessible; with free YouTube videos, online or in-person classes and options provided by charities, you have plenty of choice. You can choose from different types too, from chair yoga to highly athletic versions – it's important that you try a few classes and see how you go so you can find the one that works best for you.

There is one particular type of yoga that does not require you to move, and this is a great option for everyone, especially if you are feeling depleted and exhausted. It's called yoga nidra, or 'yogic sleep', and it is a guided meditation that promotes deep relaxation and offers other, scientifically proven, benefits.[91] It reduces stress by lowering cortisol levels, improves sleep quality and helps with relaxation. It's really amazing at helping to counter the effects of chronic stress, and also aids in emotional regulation, making it effective for managing anxiety and depression.

We have launched a wellbeing series on The Menopause and Cancer Podcast and YouTube channel, and yoga nidra is our first recording there. Try it! I've linked it in your digital handbook.

Vicky Fox is the pioneer in teaching yoga to cancer patients and author of the book *Yoga For Cancer*. Today, Vicky trains yoga teachers to teach cancer patients. She says, 'Check out a tailor-made yoga class designed specifically for cancer patients. With a specially trained instructor, you'll have someone who knows how to adjust movements to accommodate conditions like osteoporosis or lymphoedema, making the practice safer and more beneficial for you. Additionally, it comes with this great community that you can become a part of.'

If someone asks me how they can start exploring the benefits of yoga to help ease menopause symptoms, I always encourage them to ask themselves: What do you *need* right now? If you're concerned about bone health, look for classes that include strength-building elements. If stress relief and anxiety reduction are your priority, try a restorative yoga class that incorporates breathing techniques and meditation. Most yoga classes will offer a mix of benefits, so take the time to explore different styles until you find one that resonates with you. Yoga is such a versatile practice that can support you in so many ways, making it well worth the effort to find the right fit for your current needs.

Yoga has taken me on incredible journeys, from India to new friendships, and taught me mindfulness, meditation, chanting and so much more. It has had a profound impact on my life, allowing me to grow hugely as a person. It connects me to life itself. The evidence for yoga's benefits is compelling, and finding the right class could transform your experience too. Happy exploring!

Mindfulness and Meditation

Chronic stress has been linked to many health issues. Our busy lives, in which we feel stressed a lot of the time, can also intensify menopause symptoms. And of course, as many of you reading this have experienced, a cancer diagnosis and treatments add even more emotional and physical strain. Meditation and mindfulness are powerful and important evidence-based tools to counter this stress. By calming the nervous system and reducing levels of cortisol, the stress hormone linked to worsening menopause symptoms, these practices can bring much-needed relief from menopause symptoms and offer benefits for your long-term health. But of course you have to do meditation to reap its benefits, and, when life is busy and everything seems too much, one may wonder where to start.

Since my own surgical menopause, I have personally struggled with a lack of energy and tiredness for many years. Often, my days start great but by the afternoon it's hard to keep my eyes open, and I lose the ability to think clearly and concentrate. I've learned that plugging myself into a 15-minute guided meditation – I use a free one on YouTube – can help me feel refreshed and as if my whole nervous system calms down too. Being able to tap into this tool has made a huge positive impact on my daily life. In this section, I will explain some of the common misconceptions around meditation and mindfulness, some of the most common types and their benefits for cancer survivors, plus how you can make a start right away.

We have countless thoughts each day, and most of the time we're fixating on past events or worries about the future. We rarely take the time to pause and really think about what we're feeling and experiencing in the moment. By taking a moment to examine our thoughts and focus on the present, we can gain clarity, peace of mind and a sense of calm. This is the foundation of mindfulness and meditation practices.

Mindfulness and meditation are not about feeling blissed out, happy or Zen. They're not about emptying your mind or thinking about nothing. Instead, they focus on noticing what you're doing right now, acknowledging your feelings and truly meeting yourself.

Mindfulness is the practice of paying full attention to the present moment without judgement. It involves being aware of your thoughts, feelings, bodily sensations and the environment around you, and accepting them as they are. This can be very helpful if you have a tendency for your thoughts to get stuck on autopilot, so that before you know it you've been worrying over the future while doing the washing. Simple mindfulness exercises in which you focus on the present moment could include fully being aware of your actions when you are, for example, brushing your teeth, focusing on each movement, sensation in the body, sound, etc. Mindfulness can be cultivated through various other techniques too, including meditation, going on a mindful walk, breathing exercises and mindful movement practices like yoga.

I love sharing simple and practical tools with our community, and many of our workshops include mindfulness practices because they offer immediate benefits. You can practise mindfulness in several simple ways – you don't need to go anywhere or pay for a class. Try some of the below:

- Mindful breathing: focus on your breath for a few minutes. Notice the sensation of air entering and leaving your body. Perhaps notice how your chest rises and falls with your inhale and exhale. Does your belly move with your breath too? It's normal if your mind wanders. Just gently bring your focus back to your breath.

- Body scan: Developed by Jon Kabat-Zinn, this is a mindfulness practice that involves systematically focusing attention on different parts of the body. Jon Kabat-Zinn is an American professor of medicine and the creator of the Mindfulness-Based Stress Reduction (MBSR) programme (more on this below). Slow down and take your time to mentally scan your body from head to toe. Notice any areas of tension or discomfort without judgement, simply acknowledging how your body feels.

- Mindful eating: Most of us do the opposite of this when we're eating our meals, often looking at phones or watching the telly. The next time you eat, try to pay full attention to the flavours, textures and smells of your food. Eat slowly and savour each bite, noticing how it feels in your mouth.

- Walking meditation: This is my favourite. While walking, focus on the sensations of each step – the feeling of your feet touching the ground, the movement of your legs and the rhythm of your breath. Look around you. Be in awe of your surroundings. Notice the amazing world and nature.

Multiple studies have shown the benefit of how Jon Kabat-Zinn's Mindfulness-Based Stress Reduction programme can help relieve the challenging symptoms that often come with cancer and its treatments.[92] MBSR uses mindfulness practices like meditation, body scanning and gentle yoga to reduce stress. The benefits aren't just for patients currently receiving treatment; survivors also gain from it. For example, the studies show that breast cancer survivors who practised MBSR reported less anxiety, reduced fear of their cancer coming back, and improvements in physical symptoms like fatigue. Additionally, those dealing with cognitive issues related to fatigue saw lasting improvements in their quality of life.[93] For women going through menopause, MBSR can be particularly helpful as it can reduce anxiety and stress, improve mood and alleviate symptoms like fatigue. It may be worth asking your doctor if they can refer you to a programme.

Meditation is a practice where you focus your mind to achieve a state of relaxation, clarity and awareness. It involves paying attention to your breath or a specific thought, repeating a mantra or simply observing your thoughts without judgement. The goal of meditation varies; it can range from deepening self-awareness and spiritual growth to stress reduction and relaxation. Different cultures have developed their own meditation practices, each offering unique approaches, and there are many different styles of meditation, including mindfulness meditation, transcendental meditation and loving-kindness meditation, each with its own benefits.

In the early days of my yoga teacher training, I travelled to India with my yoga teacher. I was eager to be a dedicated student. Each morning, before sunrise, everyone would gather for meditation. I felt compelled to join, even though deep down I would really much have preferred to sleep in. During those hour-long meditation sessions, I was acutely aware of how uncomfortable I was. My back ached, my hips felt tight, and I couldn't stop opening my eyes for a peek to see how everyone else looked. They all seemed to be so at ease, comfortable and composed, which only made me feel more out of place. I spent a long time in those uncomfortable seated poses, questioning what I was doing and why it felt so hard. But looking back, I understand now that those early struggles were part of my growth. I was practising. This is exactly what meditation and mindfulness are – practices. You simply do them. It's not about being perfect or 'being there yet'. Many people struggle to start meditating because they think meditation requires long hours of practice or that it's only for spiritual seekers. Some also fear they won't do it 'correctly', or feel frustrated when their thoughts wander. In reality, meditation is about simply observing those thoughts without judgement, and it can be practised in short, manageable sessions.

Those early mornings in India taught me resilience and the value of persistence. They showed me that it's okay to struggle and that true practice lies in showing up even when it feels challenging. Today, I know that meditation is about being present with whatever arises, even if it's discomfort or restlessness. The good thing is, you don't need to enjoy meditating; it is still of benefit to you!

My top tip for making a start at meditation would be to listen to a guided meditation. You can download apps such as Headspace, Insight Timer and Calm, although some do come at a cost. YouTube has lots of videos that offer guided meditations too. Choose a narrating voice that you like; some come with music, others with the sounds of the sea. We have some on The Menopause and Cancer Podcast too – I've linked them in your digital handbook for you.

Journaling

Journaling is putting pen to paper and releasing some of your thoughts and emotions through the written word. You may think, 'But how is this going to help me with my menopausal symptoms?' People use journaling in different ways and for various reasons, and it can help you find some clarity. For some people, it can be a way to record specific aspects of their everyday life. For others, it's a more spontaneous exercise and a way to process experiences.

Research shows that people who use journaling have experienced reduction in depression and anxiety symptoms.[94] In her book *The Source*, neuroscientist Dr Tara Swart explains that at the very minimum journaling is a download of your emotions. She explains that 'if you keep emotions, negative thoughts or unfinished tasks in your brain–body system by thinking about them, you increase your cortisol levels, which are linked to stress. By speaking it out loud, writing it down or by embarking on physical exercise and literally sweating it out, you are releasing those negative emotions, thought patterns, anxiety and worries about the future from your brain–body system.' To me, this makes sense. Dr Latte-Naor of the Memorial Sloan Kettering Cancer Center backs it up with facts: 'A 2014 randomised controlled trial published in the prestigious *Journal of Clinical Oncology*[95] showed that expressive writing or a journaling practice led to improved cancer-related symptoms and overall physical functioning in renal cancer patients.'

It suits some people to let their words flow freely; or there are journaling practices that give you starting points: for example, you can do a simple gratitude practice where you write down a few things a day that you are grateful for. You could try this at times where you may feel 'stuck' in your menopause experience, not knowing what else you could try next to help you ease your symptoms.

A simple gratitude practice to try is to think of/write down five things that you are grateful for today. They can be anything, from having a safe home to having hot water for a cup of tea. You can be grateful for family or situations. Anything goes, however small or seemingly insignificant.

Some of the things that I might write down today include: 'I am grateful that I am able to turn on the central heating on a cold day'; 'I am grateful for the peaceful country I live in'; 'I am grateful for the cup of tea my husband just brought me'.

Numerous studies demonstrate how gratitude journaling can increase happiness.[96] One study even found that patients who expressed optimism and gratitude two weeks after an acute coronary event had healthier hearts![97] Every time a person expresses or receives gratitude, dopamine is released in the brain, therefore making a connection between the behaviour and feeling good.

At the end of each year, I host a reflection exercise and an intention-setting ceremony. You can find them on the podcast and linked in your handbook. It's a great way to get into journaling as I give prompts and it makes it very accessible. People always say how much better and more positive they feel after doing the exercise.

REFLECTIONS

Take a few moments to reflect...

1. Complementary therapies is a vast topic. From everything you have read, is there something that resonates most with you?
2. Do you want to look into accessing a particular type of therapy or trying a new supplement?
3. Make sure you are clear about your why – why you would want to tap into a therapy or take a supplement.
4. Do you need more information to do so? Such as speaking to a pharmacist or asking your doctor for a referral?

POSITIVE ACTIONS

1. What can you do for yourself today that makes you feel good? How about tuning in to a 15-minute yoga nidra for anxiety – you'll find one on our YouTube Wellbeing series.
2. Write down three things you are grateful for.
3. Healing and recovering is unique to you – there is no right or wrong. You do you.

CHAPTER 9
WHY MOVEMENT MATTERS

Exercise might seem like a small addition to what's in your menopause toolkit after cancer, but moving our bodies can be the most wonderful, impactful and accessible way for all of us to find relief from post-cancer and menopausal symptoms, plus it is proven to offer incredible benefits for your long-term health.

Physical activity does more than just get us moving; it's an essential tool that supports everything from mood stability and better sleep to stronger bones and reduced joint pain – *and* there is emerging evidence to suggest that it will help us reduce our risks of a cancer recurrence by up to 30 per cent.[98]

Whether you are able to take hormone replacement therapy (HRT) or not, and regardless of the symptoms you're experiencing, understanding how movement can support your menopausal self is crucial. Given these incredible benefits, it is a strategy that should really be prescribed to all cancer patients.

In this chapter I will share which types of exercise can help with your menopausal and post-cancer-treatment symptoms, the guidance on how much exercise is recommended post cancer and some practical tips on how you can make a start. While the research and studies I share apply to all cancer survivors, not just those experiencing menopause after treatment, I've focused on exercises that specifically help ease menopause symptoms to make it as relevant as possible for you. This chapter is not about becoming an exercise fanatic overnight. Nor will I try to convince you that one type of exercise is better than another. Instead, I want to explore with you how, bit by bit, small changes can add up to big results – so that you can draw upon exercise's healing benefits in the way that suits you and your lifestyle.

It may also be time to rethink what you consider exercise should be and discover new ways to incorporate movement into your week using approaches that are practical, manageable and still deliver real benefits. Never underestimate the power of a 20-minute walk! I'll also delve into the idea of exercise hacks to make this easier.

Take movement at your own pace; you don't need to transform everything at once. You've already been through so much, and taking back a little agency over your body can give you a sense of control. You are strong, capable and resilient, and every choice you make towards a healthy, active life is a positive step forward.

The Challenges of Movement After Cancer

Many international organisations, including the Clinical Oncology Society of Australia and the American College of Sports Medicine,[99 100] have developed exercise guidelines specifically for cancer survivors. These guidelines provide detailed recommendations, outlining not only the types of exercise but also the precise 'dose' needed to help with common post-cancer-treatment symptoms and to help reduce the risk of new cancers developing. Yet, many people I speak to ask, 'What type of exercise should I do?' and 'How much is enough to help reduce my risk of recurrence?' Or they say, 'I asked my doctors about exercise but they didn't really say much'. In fact, a 2024 survey-based study found that only 4 per cent of cancer survivors reported adhering to all four American Cancer Society (ACS) nutrition and physical activity guidelines.[101] So if you're part of the vast majority of people who had no idea these recommendations existed – you are not alone, and you're in the right place.

The authors of the study highlight that oncologists and practitioners working with cancer patients must provide more consistent and systematic guidance to encourage the adoption of healthy behaviours in this vulnerable population.[102] And I agree. We need support in addressing the lifestyle element of our recovery as much as we need support with medication or other treatments. We can't suddenly know how best to move once we're thrust into the landscape of cancer survivorship. We need to be informed and adequately supported.

Add to this the fact that bringing movement into your day can, of course, be anything but easy. You may not have exercised regularly before your cancer diagnosis, and starting now can be particularly challenging – especially if you're coping with new scars, or carrying around a suitcase full of post-treatment side effects, such as weight gain, lymphoedema, peripheral neuropathy, cardiotoxicity or fatigue. Or perhaps you don't feel as if you have the energy and stamina to do what you did before your diagnosis? Before you know it you might have cancelled one class after another out of frustration. With ongoing menopausal symptoms, just getting through the day can feel challenging at times, but I hope this chapter will inspire you to see how moving your body – whether more vigorously, or gently or mindfully – can bring renewed energy, a sense of wellbeing and menopause-symptom relief to your everyday life.

Why Movement Matters During and After Cancer Treatment

Research shows that regular exercise can play a crucial role in cancer prevention, reducing the risk of seven common types of cancer (bladder, breast, colon, endometrial, oesophageal, kidney and stomach cancers).[103 104] Additionally, it has been shown to improve survival rates and provide significant benefits for those living with cancer. It is effective in managing fatigue, enhancing overall quality of life, reducing anxiety and depression, supporting individuals affected by lymphoedema, and promoting better bone health and sleep. But please be kind to yourself when digesting this type of information. Although this is hopeful and positive data and I am sharing it to empower you, I also know many people do 'all of the right things' and still get cancer or a cancer recurrence. Cancer is never your fault. So, however much or little you moved in the past, don't blame yourself. Instead, let's use this global knowledge and years of research to our advantage, and let it help us create a lifestyle for ourselves so that we can all reap the vast benefits that exercise has to offer us.

I had the great pleasure of interviewing Professor Anna Campbell, who has spent much of her career researching the physical and psychological effects of physical activity after a cancer diagnosis. She has published over ninety research papers in the field of exercise and cancer survivorship. Today, Anna is Professor of Clinical Exercise Science at Edinburgh Napier University and director of CanRehab, and also the founder of the charity CanRehab Trust, which links people affected by cancer to trained cancer exercise specialists. When I asked Anna how she began researching the effect of movement on cancer patients, she remembered, 'Back in 2000, a friend of mine who worked with breast cancer patients told me, "Anna, I advise all my patients undergoing chemotherapy to stay in bed, to lie down, to rest, and do nothing. Is that the right message?" I replied, "Let me review the literature." After finding virtually no information about post-cancer diagnosis activities, I initiated academic research.'

Professor Campbell shared some truly eye-opening research with me: 'Evidence shows that people who don't exercise during chemotherapy experience a decline in their cardiorespiratory fitness equivalent to ageing by about ten years! However, even light activities like walking at a moderate pace most days of the week can significantly reduce that decline. We also know that women who did no strength training during chemotherapy lost muscle mass and strength similar to being in space for seven months – a common side effect of chemotherapy. But the good news is, you can prevent this decline by incorporating strength-training exercises.'

Of course, it makes sense now why so many of us struggle to get back into exercise – our cardiorespiratory fitness has declined and some of our muscles have got weaker. Additionally, Professor Campbell said that people who stay active during surgery often spend less time in the hospital and face fewer post-operative complications, which leads to a faster recovery. It was so interesting hearing this from her as I kind of felt this without knowing the facts. I didn't do anything about it when I was first diagnosed, or before or after my first surgery – I was so shell-shocked then that any thought of physical activity was totally unimaginable. But a couple of years later, when I was preparing for my double mastectomy, and, after that, for my two surgeries to remove my Fallopian tubes and later the ovaries, I felt I wanted to be in as good a physical shape as possible before my surgery. I trained hard, I ate well. I just wanted to be as fit and healthy as I could for embarking on these operations, as I felt this would help me heal and recover better. Almost as if I was preparing for my own marathon. Just as runners condition their bodies to endure the race ahead, I believed that by enhancing my physical health I would better navigate the challenges of surgery and recovery. And it turns out I was right.

Exercise is medicine

When I asked Professor Campbell whether, given all the evidence we have on the benefits of exercise, it would be wrong to suggest exercise is medicine and should be available on prescription, she replied, 'Sometimes chemotherapy drugs will only improve survival by a small percentage, whereas with exercise the emerging evidence suggests a risk reduction of up to 30 per cent.[105] While this does not mean it does completely prevent the risk of a cancer recurrence, it can lower the risk.' And of course, you have all of the benefits it brings in helping you manage symptoms as well. The tagline of the guide on moving through cancer from the American College of Sports Medicine says *Exercise Is Medicine*.[106] I'll let you make up your own mind as to what you think.

Guidelines for physical activity after cancer

So how much exercise should I do, you may ask? And what type? Here is a summary of the American Cancer Society's guidelines, which incorporate evidence-based advice on physical activity for cancer survivors:[107]

- Aim for 150–300 minutes per week of moderate-intensity activity (during which you can talk but not sing. Examples include brisk walking, yoga, leisurely bicycling, etc.).

OR

- 75–150 minutes per week of vigorous-intensity activity (during which you have trouble talking or are out of breath. Examples include running, swimming, tennis, etc.).

- OR A combination of the two intensities.

AND

- Muscle-strengthening activities two or more days per week (examples include hand weights, exercise bands and body-weight activities, such as push-ups or squats).

Given this guidance, where do we start? And how do you feel? Some of you may think, 'Well, I'm actually not far off these recommendations – great!' while others may wonder, 'Gosh, how will I ever get there?' If you have had surgery as part of your cancer treatment, you will have to be signed off by your medical team before you can start exercising.

After that, it is advised to start slowly and make sure you listen to your body. Over time, increase your exercise level to improve your fitness. Professor Campbell says, 'Even if you can only be active for a few minutes a day initially, it will help you. Slowly increase how often and how long you exercise and work towards achieving the current physical activity recommendations. The more you engage in physical activity, the greater the benefits you'll receive. So even if you're starting from a completely sedentary lifestyle and are gradually introducing some activity, you'll experience benefits. In fact, transitioning from inactivity to some activity yields more benefits than increasing activity levels from already being quite active.'

In Chapter 10, all our experts emphasise that the key to reaping benefits isn't about focusing on a single food but looking at the 'bigger picture' and what you eat over time. The same principle applies to physical activity – it's consistency and variety of movement that truly matter.

For general cancer recurrence prevention it does not matter what type of exercise you do – what matters is that you move. Each form of exercise offers unique benefits. 'Combine aerobic exercise, which raises your heart rate and breathing to improve the efficiency of your heart, lungs and circulation, with strength-building activities and stretching exercises,' advises Professor Campbell. 'Incorporate weight-bearing exercises; these don't require fancy equipment – simple moves like wall press-ups can be just as effective. The key is consistency. It's not about one individual workout but about staying active regularly over time.' Professor Campbell also reminds us of the importance of flexibility, range of motion and balance. 'For older adults, balance is particularly important. As we age, balance can decline, so practising it is vital. This is especially true for women in menopause since hormonal changes can reduce bone density, increasing the risk of fractures from falls.

Strengthening balance improves stability and coordination, helping to reduce this risk. In addition, studies have shown that if you can keep active during chemotherapy it helps reduce weight gain, which can often happen during cancer treatment.'

On page 233, I'll guide you through creating your very own 'exercise plan'. This will help you choose from a variety of wonderful movement options to craft a plan that suits your abilities, energy levels and lifestyle. As Professor Campbell advises, 'Focus on these key elements – cardiovascular fitness, strength, flexibility and balance – and aim for consistency. That's what makes the biggest difference.'

Wherever you are right now as you read this, honour your starting point. Each of you is at a different stage in your journey, with unique histories when it comes to exercise. Some of you may feel energised and motivated to try new activities, while others might find even a 10-minute walk challenging – and that's okay. I can't stress this enough: it's not about where you've been but about where you go from here. What truly matters is how you choose to move forward from today.

Help to get started

Professor Campbell echoes what I believe to be important to set ourselves up for success. 'Remember, you don't have to do this all by yourself, ' she says. Professor Campbell took time out of academia to set up CanRehab. They train physiotherapists, personal trainers, doctors and nurses, and anyone else aiming to help people affected with cancer, to give evidence-based and safe expert advice on exercise and rehabilitation. It may be helpful to consult a cancer exercise specialist to create a fitness plan that's suited to your needs.

Sarah Newman, a wonderful lady who ran a strength-training for cancer survivors webinar for us at Menopause and Cancer, is a cancer exercise specialist. After being diagnosed with a gynaecological cancer at the age of 28 and while pregnant, Sarah navigated through treatments feeling uncertain about which type of exercise she could do safely. 'Despite feeling rubbish during treatment, I wanted to move more during recovery, but I was unsure about what to do and what was safe,' she says. 'Initially I joined a post-natal class for pelvic floor and core strength, which did help, but as you can imagine, that was completely the wrong setting for me. I then transitioned to basic yoga, resistance training and cardiovascular exercises and so I gradually rebuilt my strength.' Encouraged by her own journey and using her background in science, she delved into becoming a cancer and exercise specialist herself. 'I want to help others find a path to recovery and strength,' says Sarah, who has since founded Get Me Back, an online platform that provides clear and specialist advice on fitness and nutrition specifically for women affected by cancer.

There are many other great initiatives you could look up. Move Against Cancer is a charity that leads an initiative called 5K Your Way to support people to run, walk or jog five kilometres at their local park run. If you're in the UK, you can connect to charities such as Macmillan, Maggie's and Trekstock. Regardless of whether you have never exercised in the past, or have been an avid-gym goer and that's changed, it's okay. If you think a structured plan and some support in getting you going are what you need, reach out to organisations that can help you.

How exercise can help with post-cancer and menopause symptom relief

Research shows that, for certain side effects, there is enough evidence to recommend specific exercise prescriptions to help alleviate symptoms. These prescriptions focus on four key components: frequency, intensity, duration and type. However, as Professor Anna Campbell of Edinburgh Napier University and CanRehab explains, 'Not everyone needs to start at the recommended level. It's perfectly fine to begin at your own pace and gradually build up over time.'

Fatigue

As anyone in that position knows, fatigue after cancer is a uniquely persistent, overwhelming exhaustion. It can be compounded by menopause and the lack of hormones. Sleep disturbances, which as we have seen are common, and the additional emotional stress can make fatigue much worse. Professor Campbell told me: 'Once you've had your surgery and if you're beginning chemotherapy or radiotherapy, one of the biggest issues we've found is cancer-related fatigue. The evidence from around seventy studies strongly indicates that staying active can mitigate this fatigue.'

While it may seem counterintuitive to move when you're tired, women have reported reduced fatigue and improved sleep levels after engaging in physical activities. Research supports this, showing that exercise and psychological interventions are highly effective for reducing cancer-related fatigue (CRF) both during and after cancer treatment, often outperforming available pharmaceutical options.[108]

There is strong evidence to show that the following types and doses of exercise help:

- Aerobic exercise only: 3x/week for 30 min per session of moderate intensity.
- Resistance exercise only: 2x/week of 2 sets of 12–15 reps for major muscle groups at moderate intensity.
- Combination (Aerobic + Resistance): 3x/week for 30 min per session of moderate aerobic exercise, plus 2x/week of resistance training 2 sets of 12–15 reps for major muscle groups at moderate intensity.[109]

Anxiety

Anxiety is a common symptom of the menopause, and it is of course very common in cancer survivors experiencing induced menopause. The emotional impact of cancer treatment, hormonal changes and our worries about the future, together with the challenges of managing other ongoing menopausal symptoms, can make anxiety a persistent companion for so many of us. Alongside the other strategies that I list in the Symptom Troubleshooter (see pages 274–277), exercise can help by reducing stress hormones, boosting endorphins, improving mood and promoting relaxation, all of which can help improve anxiety. In Chapter 9, I also discuss in detail how yoga has helped me manage anxiety and the positive impact it has had on my mental health.

Research suggests that the following type and dose of exercise can help with managing anxiety:

- Aerobic exercise only: 3x/week for 30–60 min per session of moderate to vigorous intensity.

- Combination (Aerobic + Resistance): 2–3x/week for 20–40 min of moderate to vigorous aerobic exercise, plus 2x/week of resistance training of 2 sets, 8–12 reps for major muscle groups at moderate to vigorous intensity.[110]

Note that, for anxiety, there is so far insufficient evidence to indicate that resistance exercise on its own has notable benefits.

Low mood and depression

Most of us will have heard that exercise is a good mood booster, helping us to feel better, and many talk about that 'exercise high' they experience after working out. Yet, often the last thing we feel like doing when we're feeling low or depressed is move. This can, in turn, make us feel guilty for not doing enough, and so the negative cycle of inactivity continues. So whatever you can do to avoid inactivity is great. Even working towards the recommendations will be of benefit to your mood. Encourage yourself to go for a 15-minute walk in the morning, open your eyes to the daylight and watch the world wake up. I have not heard many people say that they felt worse after a walk. Remember, any movement is beneficial.

Research suggests that the following type and dose of exercise can help with managing low mood and depression:

- Aerobic exercise only: 3x/week for 30–60 minutes per session of moderate to vigorous intensity.

- Combination (Aerobic + Resistance): 2–3x/week for 20–40 minutes of moderate to vigorous aerobic exercise, plus 2x/week of resistance training of 2 sets, 8–12 reps for major muscle groups at moderate to vigorous intensity.[111]

Note that, for low mood and depression, there is so far insufficient evidence to indicate that resistance exercise on its own has notable benefits.

Osteoporosis/osteopenia

Cancer treatments and menopause, particularly early menopause, can have a significant negative impact on bone health, increasing the risk of osteopenia and osteoporosis. The drop in oestrogen levels, the key hormone for maintaining bone density, accelerates bone loss, especially in women who enter menopause prematurely due to cancer treatments. Additionally, women on hormone blockers, such as aromatase inhibitors, experience further oestrogen suppression, compounding this effect. These factors can lead to weakened bones, making fractures more likely. Rebekah Rotstein, the founder of BUFF BONES®, which trains midlife women as well as exercise professionals for better bone and joint health, explains, 'Despite current diagnoses based on bone density scores from a DEXA scan, osteoporosis technically is not just low bone density but also changes in the bone structure and architecture that make it more likely to fracture. A DEXA scan is a medical imaging test used to measure bone mineral density, which helps to assess the risk of fractures and diagnose conditions like osteoporosis.'

Some experts say that for women osteoporosis is 'the silent killer' – which can make us feel utterly hopeless and defeated. Exercise, however, alongside diet and the other strategies I mention on pages 301–304, can make a huge difference in helping us look after our bone health going forward.

Since I know that bone loss is a huge worry for many of the people in our community, I wanted to go into more detail here, to fully empower you with the knowledge you need so that you know exactly what type of exercise can help you build better bones. Rebekah Rotstein says, 'Because cancer treatment can compromise bone quality, it's helpful to seek the expertise of a professional with knowledge in exercise for bone health. For example, certain motions, like sit-ups (rounding the back against gravity or with the entire body weight loaded on the rounded back) could increase a spine fracture in someone who's undergone treatment and has osteoporosis or osteopenia. Focus on building muscle mass as this is protective to the skeleton. When it comes to bone density, weight-bearing exercise with strength training is key, along with the impact training. High-intensity exercise, at a level that challenges you, may have the best potential to improve bone density, but it's important to gradually work up to this, especially for those who've undergone cancer treatment. For instance, start off learning to hinge at the hips, keeping your back straight, like when picking up a heavy box. Over time, add more weight to the box so that eventually you can pick up something quite heavy. Technique matters, of course, but this and exercises like squats and lunges are essential for better bones. Additionally, training balance and power help prevent falls and fractures and should be included in your exercise programme for bone health. There are so many ways to train your body to prevent fractures. Our bodies and bones are exceptionally adaptive. It's never too late to get started.'

Brain health

Most of us reading this will have experienced ourselves that brain health can be negatively affected by menopause, especially early menopause.

Memory problems, difficulty concentrating – the dreaded brain fog. Additionally, research suggests that early menopause may increase the risk of neurodegenerative conditions like Alzheimer's disease later in life due to prolonged oestrogen deficiency.[112] Dr Lisa Mosconi, a neuroscientist, pioneering authority and researcher on women's brain health, and author of the brilliant book *The Menopause Brain*, explains how exercise can positively affect women going through menopause by supporting brain health. Her findings show that exercise plays a critical role in mitigating some of the most common menopause symptoms by boosting brain energy levels, enhancing the brain's ability to use glucose, and potentially slowing down neurodegeneration processes linked to Alzheimer's. Physical activity may help reduce stress in the brain, improve mood and support cognitive function, making it an essential tool for women who are experiencing menopausal symptoms.

A Holistic Exercise Strategy

Since it's most important to me that we approach our health and address menopausal symptoms in a holistic and, most importantly, doable and practical way, I wanted to share an example of how different strategies can each play a unique role. Dr Annice Mukherjee highlights in her book, *The Complete Guide to the Menopause*, that chronic stress can negatively impact bone health over time. This is why it's so important to include a variety of movement strategies in our toolbox – each of them contributes in its own way, and you can add and use them at a pace that feels right for you. Exercises like yoga and mindfulness are excellent for stress reduction and can complement other activities, like weight training. If you're not ready to take on weight-lifting yet, remember that lowering your stress levels can positively impact your bone and overall health too. Don't put yourself off by thinking that you need to do it all at once. Instead, focus on recognising the deep connection between your physical, mental and emotional health, and understand that different types of exercise can uniquely support various aspects of your wellbeing. Exercise is profoundly powerful, and it doesn't have to be an either/or approach – it's about finding what works best for you right now, one step at a time.

Your Exercise Plan

You need a plan that works for you. Think about it this way: just as a doctor prescribes medication, it's now your turn to prescribe your own movement plan.

1. Start by tallying up how much you currently move each week. Be honest!

2. Compare your current activity levels to the guidance provided provided in the previous pages and identify any areas where you are falling short. You might be starting from scratch by working towards 30 minutes of walking most days. Or you might be pleasantly surprised to find that you're doing better than you thought you are. Or you might discover that you need to add some strength- training.

3. Plan how you will incorporate the movement element that's missing. Are you going to join an in-person local group class? Will you sign up to an online course? Will you plan in a weekly walk with your friends? Will you reach out to a charity to ask what's on offer? Remember, if you fail to plan, you are planning to fail.

4. Now write down your exercise prescription and put the activities into your diary, even if it is just to plan in that 15-minute morning walk. This will hopefully make it easier for you to stick to it.

My Top Five Tips to Make Movement Part of Your Daily Life

As with many things in life, you might be feeling motivated to move at first, but I want to gently remind you that your motivation may dwindle at times; we can't always rely on motivation to achieve what we set out to do. Many of your menopause symptoms will change over time, and it can be hard to stick to the best of plans when they seem to be wanting to take over. So in addition to your exercise plan, I have a few other tips that I want to give you to help try to ensure you stick to it.

The first is **'move with joy'**. When you truly connect to a form of movement that you enjoy, you can't really go wrong, and it will help keep you going.

The second is **'explore'**. The you today is different to the pre-cancer you – so the way you enjoy moving may be different too. You might have to go on a little journey of discovery about what type of movement you enjoy now, and you might have to spur yourself on to try some new things. It can take some courage to try out a new Zumba class, or to give your local Parkrun a go, but you'll never know what's out there and what you might be missing unless you try! Start swimming, bouldering, yoga, rollerblading, hiking, Pilates, weight-lifting classes, barre classes, strength classes, tennis, cycling, table tennis, badminton, trampolining... Go for it! Seek out the joy, and you might find it right round the corner, whether it's in your morning stroll or a style of dance you'd never imagined yourself loving.

The third tip is to incorporate **'exercise snacks'** into your day. The evidence Professor Anna Campbell of Edinburgh Napier University and CanRehab outlined earlier didn't state that you need to do hour-long sessions to gain the benefits of moving. And perhaps by adding shorter segments of movement into your days you will be able to reach the recommended guidance without too many problems.

A wonderful dietician, Elizabeth Ward, once told me, 'Surprise your bones, Dani!' And what she meant was 'mix things up'. Since then, I almost always jump down the last few stairs. It might sound like a weird thing to do, but it's great for my bones, plus it gives me a moment of joy too. Many people in the wellbeing space recommend exercise snacks because the concept really does help us stay active throughout the day, even if we do not have time for a full one-hour class at the gym. Try standing on one leg while brushing your teeth, or doing some wall press-ups every now and then, and you'll see how effective this is, or maybe even addictive. It's such a good feeling to move little and often. My friend Dinah Siman is a brilliant Pilates instructor; I follow her on Instagram, where she shares many of her exercise snacks with her audience. You'll often find me squatting before or even after a walk or run; and I really do flip myself into a downward dog waiting while my spaghetti water boils. I am so sure that it helps me feel well.

My fourth tip is **'be kind to yourself'**. Some days will be harder than others, and that's okay. If you're tired or dealing with menopausal symptoms, focus on small, gentle movements rather than intense workouts. Listen to your body and celebrate every little bit of effort – whether it's a slow stretch or a quick walk. And on some days it might be that gentle meditation is the exercise you need for your mind.

And my fifth tip is to **'find a buddy or community'**. Exercising with others can make a huge difference. The social element adds accountability and fun, making it so much easier to stay consistent. Even online communities or virtual classes can offer a sense of connection and support. I know that all the people who join my wonderful friend Vicky Fox's online yoga for cancer classes gain so much from the sense of belonging they experience.

Move together: Menopause and cancer in action

The incredible benefits of exercise have been pretty clear to me for a long time, but the numerous obstacles and hurdles many of us face in actually sticking to it are not lost on me either. I've always wanted to find ways of encouraging all the women in our community to move in ways that are fun and bring them joy. So our Menopause and Cancer organisation has hosted a variety of walking challenges in which everyone could take part, anywhere in the world. People set their own goals – because of course we all have different levels of fitness – and we each decided if we wanted to commit to walking every day or if we wanted to train up for a big walk. We even hosted longer marathon-walk fundraising challenges. We had women from all over lace up their shoes and head out walking through the seasons, come rain or shine. Some walked together in groups, and others walked alone and found that really cathartic. So, let this encourage you to seek out your community. Join a class, find a workout partner, or look for local walking, running or cycling groups – or perhaps even sign yourself up for a charity challenge. It is powerful to do things as a community and it can bring you so many rewards.

REFLECTIONS

Take a few moments to reflect...

1. How much did you move before your cancer diagnosis?
2. How much physical activity do you do currently?
3. Compare how far off you are from the current guidelines for physical activity – or are you meeting the requirements?

POSITIVE ACTIONS

1. How can you move today in ways to make you feel good?
2. Which type of movement brings you joy? Or, if you're just starting out, explore what that could be.
3. Moving with friends and a supportive community can be so much better than going it alone – pick up the phone and ask a friend to join you for a walk and a natter.
4. Who is going to support you? Don't make it vague – plan where you are going to do your exercise. When are you going to do it? Plan for what to do during the holidays, or how to get back into it after a period of being more sedentary.
5. Download your digital handbook if you have not already done so – I have included lots of helpful exercise links for you.

CHAPTER 10
WHAT YOU EAT MATTERS

Diet is a powerful tool within the range of lifestyle options available to help manage menopausal symptoms. What you eat not only plays a key role in alleviating these symptoms but also supports long-term health and helps reduce the risk of cancer recurrence. In my opinion, the way we eat can become one of our most supportive daily strategies, making us an active participant in our recovery process, our healing and continued wellbeing. I know it is such a privilege to be able to eat well, one that I believe can not only have a positive impact on our physical health but on our mental health too.

But of course, diet is also one of the most complex strategies to tackle, because, if eating healthily was easy, wouldn't we all be sitting in front of perfectly balanced plates three times a day?

When I was going through active cancer treatment my mother-in-law bought me a book on how diet can help ease chemotherapy side effects, such as mouth ulcers, diarrhoea and constipation, and this was the first time I had thought, *I wonder what else food can do for me?* Although I come from a home in which my own mum always prepared wonderful meals for us, as an adult I had not been paying attention to what I ate at all. I was living off salami sandwiches and ready meals. When everyone else ate one slice of cake, I'd often have two, and there was a reason why people called me the 'Schnapps queen' – and it wasn't just because I am Austrian! Yet one of the first things I wanted to change after my diagnosis was the food I consumed.

Admittedly, initially my main focus was on what I should remove from my diet, as I thought that by cutting out certain foods I could reduce my risks of a cancer recurrence. So I cut out all sugars, alcohol, meat, wheat, dairy, anything ready made and animal products overnight. Today I understand that much of my drastic action was driven by fear of recurrence and the many myths surrounding diet and cancer. Plus, it was most likely also a way of clawing back some of the control cancer had swiped. Between then and today lies a long journey of transformation. I have gone on a real quest to nourish myself and my family to the best of my ability. I went on many detours, experimented in my own kitchen and, as I studied nutrition in more detail, my diet became 'full-of' rather than 'free-from'. All of this led me to making many U-turns in how I ate, adapting to the many changes and needs of my body; today I call this my very own food revolution. By the time I entered surgical menopause I was confident that the way I ate would support my menopausal self alongside the other strategies I outline in this book. I also knew diet would support my bones, brain and heart in the long run. Paying attention to my diet felt empowering – knowing I could fuel my body to help support it after everything it had gone through. Alongside my yoga practice, food did become my medicine and an integral part of my support toolbox. Besides, eating well gave me back so much hope and gratitude – hope that I was on the right track; gratitude for each meal and every day.

How You Eat Is Very Personal

Of course, you will have your own history with food, and diet may or may not be something you want to address right now. How we eat and how we feel about how we eat is a highly personal thing. Registered nutritional therapist Julie Webb is somebody I have worked with for a number of years, and she explained to me that my own experience resembles that of many patients she has been helping over the years, saying, 'I have seen cancer patients for over seventeen years and, by the time they come and see me for nutritional advice, the chances are that they are anxious about their diet and have already made some dietary changes or cut some foods out.'

I love Julie's non-judgemental and practical approach, and I am grateful that she has shared many of her hands-on tips with us in this chapter. She says, 'Maybe you're eating so much broccoli you're wondering whether you might turn green! Maybe you feel your diet is already pretty healthy, but you are still thinking, *What else can I do?* Or perhaps, like the majority of clients I have seen, you are feeling overwhelmed and confused about what you can safely eat now. You may want to know which foods to eat to help manage your menopause symptoms. Or perhaps you may be wanting to know which foods to avoid to help prevent a recurrence of your cancer?'

In short, everyone reading this may have a different concern or question, and so I thought long and hard about how to tackle this chapter. I wanted to address the many common concerns that have been raised by our community at the workshops I have run with dietitians, nutritionists and researchers.

I will include advice from a variety of experts. Julie Webb will share her practical insights on what makes a balanced plate to help reduce menopause symptoms, alongside advice on how diet can help address them. You will also be hearing from Professor Sarah Berry, a professor in the Department of Nutritional Sciences at King's College London and chief scientist at ZOE. Sarah will help us look at the latest research on diet and menopause. And I will also share with you the current cancer prevention guidance on diet for cancer survivors, which includes what not to eat after cancer.

As with the other chapters, this is general advice. Some readers may have unique dietary needs. For instance, if you've been advised to follow a low-fibre diet after bowel cancer treatment, much of this advice here may not be suitable for you. Be sure to consult a cancer dietitian, registered dietitian or registered nutritional therapist for guidance tailored to your recovery and specific needs.

Is There a Diet That's Best for Menopausal Symptoms?

One of the biggest mistakes I see people make is that they don't quite believe their diet can have a profound impact on their menopausal symptoms. 'We know that eating a typical Western diet, which is high in ultra-processed foods, refined sugars, unhealthy fats, processed meats, and low in fruits, vegetables and whole grains, is linked to several health problems. Research is showing that such a diet can contribute to conditions like obesity, Type 2 diabetes, cardiovascular diseases and certain cancers,' explains Julie Webb.

She continues, 'On the other hand, research shows that the Mediterranean diet promotes healthier ageing, offering benefits like a longer life expectancy, reduced chronic disease, lower cancer rates and improved heart health.[113] I'll explain exactly what the Mediterranean diet is in more detail later on, but know that by adopting this approach you can also reduce the risk of developing Type 2 diabetes, high blood pressure and cholesterol issues, which are all conditions that increase after menopause and early menopause after cancer in particular. Studies even suggest it may help protect against neurological conditions, such as Alzheimer's.[114] Again, I know this is a worry for many women in menopause after cancer. Some of my clients even worry that their brain fog is the early onset of dementia. Additionally, we know the Mediterranean diet is linked to better bone health, which is also a concern for most of my clients.'

When I asked Julie if she thought it was really possible to reduce one's menopause symptoms by eating a Mediterranean-style diet she was quick to say, 'Absolutely! I see it happen all the time and research also tells us so.[115] Women tell me symptoms such as joint ache, fatigue, sleep disturbances and hot flushes improve significantly. But it is not about relying on adding lots of one particular food or removing another altogether. It is the bigger picture and the variety of foods you eat over time that is going to make the biggest difference.'

Sarah Berry of King's College London and ZOE is at the forefront of studying the impact of diet on women. I asked her what their latest research on diet and the impact on menopause symptoms showed and she explained, 'Historically, most trials have focused on men, partly because male participants are simpler to analyse because you don't have to account for hormonal fluctuations. But I am delighted to be able to confirm that our latest, and much-needed, research results for women are in.'

She went on, 'Many studies have explored supplements and individual foods with inconsistent results, so I don't believe any single food or nutrient is universally effective. But there is strong evidence that an overall healthy dietary pattern can help manage menopause symptoms. There's no single "magic bullet" solution, but studies consistently show that following a Mediterranean-style diet or a balanced diet rich in plant-based whole foods, high in fibre and polyphenols, and with minimal ultra-processed foods, sugar and salt can significantly alleviate symptoms. This overall approach to healthy eating is beneficial for all adults – male, female, pre- or postmenopausal. Recently, we published an abstract that explored menopause symptom reduction through the ZOE personalised nutrition programme, which focuses on dietary improvements. We evaluated diet quality with the Healthy Eating Index (HEI), finding that higher HEI scores, which reflect healthier diets, were inversely related to the severity of menopausal symptoms. This means that individuals who scored higher in diet quality reported fewer symptoms.

'Additionally, we tracked symptom changes before and after the ZOE personalised nutrition programme and observed up to a 35 per cent symptom reduction, as measured by a tool called the Menoscale. This scale quantifies both the frequency of menopause symptoms and their impact on quality of life. Even small improvements in the quality of your diet can lead to noticeable relief from menopause symptoms. In other words, if you make gradual changes to eat healthier, you may feel better and experience fewer symptoms.'

This is fantastic news! We urgently need more research focused on women's health and it's not only encouraging to see this starting to happen, but also exciting that the latest findings show how dietary choices can positively impact our experiences.

You are worth your time and energy

The second-biggest mistake I see people make is that they don't feel they are worthy of the time and energy it takes to tackle their diet. I am sure we can all agree that to make eating healthily a habit, there will inevitably be a bit of planning, ingredient shopping, prepping and then cooking, all before we even get to do the eating. After I had changed my own way of eating I started to get so many questions from other mums on the school run: How do you manage to eat so well with three little ones? So what is it you eat if you don't eat meat? etc. – and so I founded the SuperFood SupperClub, which involved groups of people coming to my house to cook delicious recipes together, with the aim of showing them that healthy eating can be easy, affordable *and* tasty. At the end of our cooking sessions we all sat down and ate together, which was the highlight of each event for me. That was when most people shared that they made much more effort for everyone else and that their own dietary needs often came last. Women in particular prioritised their offspring and other halves, often making extravagant packed lunches while they mindlessly reached for a packet of biscuits instead of eating a nourishing meal. And if it wasn't children that took that priority spot, it was their job, hobbies and other duties that meant there was little time and energy left to prep and cook good food for themselves. The biggest compliment I often received was, 'Wow, I love that you look after yourself so well!' And I really did and still do. I feel I deserve good food; I deserve to make an effort for myself. I deserve the joy eating with my family and friends gives me. And I am very grateful that I have access to good food.

This does not mean I eat a super-healthy diet all the time. It means I eat well a lot of the time, and that's what matters. Julie says, 'The good news is that, while each of you is unique in terms of how you need to nourish your body, diet doesn't need to be hard and it doesn't have to be (and never can be) perfect. We have to let go of judgement and blame right from the start. To me, there is absolutely no room for either of those in nutrition. After a diagnosis and treatment, many patients feel highly motivated to change their eating habits. However, this motivation can fade over time, and old habits may creep back in. Sometimes, changes aren't made consistently, leading to ongoing anxiety about diet and feelings of guilt with every meal. This is why I believe it's important for motivation to come from how *food makes you feel* and let those benefits be what motivate you, rather than fear. The most important but the hardest thing of all is sticking to a less processed diet in our busy and complex world surrounded by convenience foods.'

Acknowledge and celebrate your efforts and be kind to yourself on the days when your meals just did not go as planned.

If your main takeaway from this chapter is to focus on eating fewer processed foods and remember that you deserve to invest time and energy into making positive changes for yourself, then you're already off to a great start. Small, sustainable and intentional steps can set the foundation for a healthier, more empowered you.

Your Menopause Diet Explained

Rather than a strict diet, the Mediterranean diet represents a style of eating inspired by traditional food practices in Mediterranean coastal regions, including countries like Italy, Greece, Turkey, Spain and France. Unlike the many diets that focus on short-term goals such as weight loss or muscle building, the Mediterranean diet emphasises healthy eating habits as a sustainable, lifelong approach. Julie says, 'I want to encourage you not to pin all your hopes on an extra serving of broccoli now and again, but instead look at the bigger picture. Take some time to note what you're eating over the period of a week and then compare how far off you are from the Mediterranean style of eating. That's always a good starting point. You can then create a plan to gradually incorporate more elements of the Mediterranean diet into your meals.'

To help ease menopause symptoms and to support your long-term health, we will focus on several key areas, including ensuring you consume enough dietary fibre to stabilise blood-sugar levels and nourish your gut bacteria. It's also important to incorporate adequate amounts of protein into each meal and to ensure sufficient vegetable and calcium intake to support bone health. And if you are wondering if dietary recommendations are different for menopause and for cancer survivors, don't worry! I cover the cancer prevention guidelines in much detail as well.

The Mediterranean diet focuses on a variety of plant-based foods like vegetables, fruits and whole grains (such as wholegrain rice, barley, spelt, oats and quinoa), complemented by healthy fats mainly from olive oil, avocados, nuts and seeds. It encourages regular portions of legumes for protein and fibre, as well as moderate amounts of fish, particularly oily fish, such as salmon and mackerel, for heart-healthy omega-3s. Dairy, such as yoghurt and cheese, and poultry are included, while red meat and refined sugars are limited.

Your Menopause Plate

To turn the idea of the Mediterranean diet into a practical way of eating, Julie suggests starting by looking at your plate. 'It can be really helpful to visualise how much of each food group should feature in your meals. This gives you a practical guide and means you will not have to weigh out foods, which I am not a fan of as it makes eating difficult and people get too caught up in the smaller details,' she explains. Julie also recommends eating three meals a day within a 12-hour window. 'This is a good way to ensure you eat a balanced intake of all the essential nutrients you need for your recovery, to help manage menopausal symptoms and support your body's needs during this challenging time. Of course you can eat two meals a day, but as we go through the next steps you will see that this might not give you enough of an opportunity to nourish yourself fully,' she explains.

So what does a balanced menopause plate look like?

The nourishing half

Aim for half a plate of fruit and vegetables at each meal. This helps support digestion and provides essential fibre, vitamins and minerals. 'You might be thinking this sounds like more than the typical UK guidelines of a "five-a-day" goal,' says Julie. 'Many clients feel this is challenging, and that's completely normal. If you're not reaching this yet, don't worry. The key is to work towards this goal gradually, at a pace that suits you. It's not about perfection but about making small, consistent steps. Don't worry about the sugar content of fruit; in its whole form fruit is perfectly fine and adds a wonderful variety of nutrients. Aim for three servings a day.'

The benefits of consuming a variety of fruits and vegetables extend beyond overall health and significantly impact menopause symptoms. Here are some key benefits:

Fibre

Fibre is essential for managing menopause symptoms because it supports your gut health, aids in weight management and promotes stable blood-sugar levels, which can reduce hot flushes and mood swings.[116 117] You also need plenty of fibre to keep your heart healthy, and dietary fibre has been associated with a lower risk of certain types of cancer, particularly colorectal cancer. The UK government recommends eating 30g of fibre per day. Unfortunately, most people don't meet this goal.[118]

In practice, you could be smashing your fibre goals if you ate the following over the course of a day:

- ½ large avocado contains about 8g of fibre
- ½ tin of kidney beans contains about 11.5g
- 1 x 75g serving of wholemeal pasta contains 8g
- 1 medium apple contains about 4.5g
- 1 medium pear contains about 6g

Antioxidants, vitamins and minerals

Minerals such as magnesium and calcium are essential for muscle and nerve function, as well as bone health, and it is crucial that we support this as we know that menopause, and especially early menopause, has a negative impact on bone density.

Sources of magnesium include flaxseed, chia seeds, nuts and green leafy veg.

Good sources of calcium include milk, cheese and other dairy products; green leafy veg, such as curly kale, okra, but not spinach (spinach does contain high levels of calcium but the body cannot digest it all), plant-based milks with added calcium; bread and anything made with fortified flour.

Fruit and vegetables, such as berries, beetroot, spinach and raw cacao, also deliver antioxidants that will help you combat oxidative stress.[119] Increased oxidative stress can exacerbate menopause symptoms, including hot flushes and mood swings, and is linked to chronic conditions such as cardiovascular disease, osteoporosis, cancer, anxiety and depression.

Polyphenols

Polyphenols are naturally occurring compounds found in fruits, vegetables, coffee, tea and other plant-based foods such as spices, and they are known for their significant anti-cancer benefits.[120] Research also indicates that polyphenols may offer significant benefits for managing arthralgia – this is the medical term for joint ache – through their anti-inflammatory properties. Eating plenty of fruit and vegetables will provide you with the wonderful benefit of polyphenols. Vegetables rich in polyphenols are spinach, kale, red onions and artichokes. Legumes and beans are great sources of polyphenols too, as are nuts, seeds, dark chocolate, whole grains and fruit, especially red grapes. Tea and coffee contain polyphenols too.

My top tips to add more fruit and veg into your day

- Have a packet of frozen vegetables such as spinach or peas in your freezer – they're great for throwing into a pasta sauce or a stew, so that you've got a portion of veg ready to go.

- Frozen fruit, such as berries, make a quick and nutritious addition to your breakfast.

- Add mild-tasting veggies like spinach or cucumber to a smoothie.

- When you make your breakfast in the morning, prepare yourself a veggie snack, such as some carrots cut up and ready for dipping in hummus, or celery sticks to have with peanut butter, for the afternoon or when energy levels are low. The key is in the prep; if it's ready to go, you won't find yourself reaching for something more convenient but less healthy.

The energising half

To fully support your overall health and wellbeing, and to help ease menopausal symptoms, you need to complement the *nourishing half* of your plate with the *energising half*. This half is your opportunity to include complex carbohydrates (starches), protein and healthy fats in each of your meals. These are known as essential macronutrients and they play a crucial role in maintaining energy levels, supporting bone health and promoting cardiovascular health during menopause, among many other essential functions. For example:

- Complex carbohydrates provide steady energy and help stabilise blood-sugar levels, which is going to be key in helping you combat fatigue.

- Protein is essential for muscle mass maintenance and repair; it also promotes satiety, which is helpful in weight management during menopause.

- Healthy fats contribute to heart health and help reduce inflammation, which in return can help with joint aches and pains.

Julie says, 'These food groups cause people the most concern. People worry about carbs and their potential impact on weight or blood-sugar levels. Protein is another macronutrient that raises questions. "Can I eat meat?" or "I know soy is a good source of protein, but I am not sure I can have it as I had a hormone-sensitive cancer," are just a couple of the comments I hear over and over again.'

We'll address these concerns later on (see page 252), but for now, remember to work towards creating this balanced plate[121] for most of your meals so that you can enhance your body's functioning, reduce menopause symptoms and help prevent chronic disease.

Protein

'The media have done a pretty good job of making sure we are all aware that menopausal women should be eating more protein,' Julie tells me. Consuming adequate amounts of protein offers several significant benefits, from preserving lean muscle, which is vital for maintaining strength, and improving bone density, all the way to helping you stay fuller for longer. For cancer survivors it is also important to point out that adequate protein intake can support recovery and your immune system. Additionally, cancer treatments can lead to muscle wastage, making protein intake even more important for maintaining muscle mass and strength during recovery. Julie explains, 'Many women with a history of cancer come to see me reporting that they've gone plant-based since their diagnosis. However, many have not fully adjusted their diets to include enough plant-based protein sources in place of animal proteins, which can leave them falling short of an adequate protein intake.'

How much protein do I need?

The recommended nutrient intake from the UK government is to eat 0.75g of protein per kilogram of body weight per day. So if you weigh 65kg, you'd be aiming to eat around 48g of protein a day. The World Cancer Research Fund recommends consuming between 1 and 1.5g of protein a day per kilogram of body weight during cancer treatment.[122] Requirements are higher during treatment to help your body to repair and regenerate. If you weigh 65kg, this would be between 65g and 98g per day.

The following might help you work towards your goals:

- 1 x 175g raw chicken breast contains about 55g protein
- 1 (approx. 100g) raw salmon fillet contains about 22g protein
- 150g tofu contains about 24g protein
- 150g Greek yoghurt contains about 13.5g protein
- 20g shelled hemp seeds contain about 6.7g protein

It is important that you achieve the recommended dietary allowance (RDA) for protein but, with so much emphasis on eating protein throughout menopause, many of us can get fixated on filling our plates with protein at the expense of other important dietary requirements, such as fibre. More is not better; you just need enough.

Protein is found in a large variety of foods, whatever your dietary preferences:

Animal foods rich in protein include meat (beef, pork, poultry), fish and seafood, eggs and dairy products (milk, yoghurt, cheese).

Plant-based protein sources include soybeans (tofu, tempeh and edamame), lentils, chickpeas, black beans, kidney beans, peas, quinoa, hemp seeds, chia seeds, pumpkin seeds, almonds, walnuts, brown rice, oats, and even spinach.

Protein powders can be a quick way to increase your protein intake. Check the ingredients list and avoid added sugars, artificial sweeteners and fillers. A short list of recognisable ingredients is typically a good sign.

My top tips to add protein into your day

- For breakfasts, sprinkle shelled hemp seeds over a bowl of full-fat yoghurt or kefir with fruits, nuts and seeds. It's often the combination of foods that will give you the recommended amount of protein, not a single food itself.

- For main meals, try adding split red lentils to pasta sauces and stews; they dissolve and have a very mild taste. Add a tin of cannellini beans or a handful of cashews to soups; they make it super creamy when you blitz it.

Carbohydrates

Julie says, 'Poor old carbohydrates have had such a bad press over the last few years with the rise of keto diets and low-carb eating for weight loss. And so many of my clients come to me saying they have cut out sugar and carbs completely and present a food diary that is both insufficient and unsustainable. The simple solution is not to cut out carbs completely but to choose your carbs wisely. Complex carbohydrates (as opposed to simple carbohydrates) are generally rich in fibre, vitamins and minerals, making them beneficial for your health. Choose wholegrain and unrefined carbohydrates such as brown rice, quinoa and oats. Add legumes, such as beans and lentils, and starchy vegetables like sweet potatoes and corn. Include wholegrain bread and pasta. These complex carbohydrates are digested more slowly than simple, refined carbohydrates, which means that they provide a gradual release of glucose into the bloodstream that helps to maintain stable energy levels and prevent large spikes in blood sugar. There's no need to avoid gluten unless you are coeliac. A serving of carbs with your evening meal can also help with sleep.'

My top tip to add complex carbs into your day

- Make my staple three-bean salad once a week, then have it as a side with your protein and veg, or ladle over a jacket sweet potato boat for an easy lunch or snack on it in the afternoon. To make the salad, drain and rinse three 400g tins of different varieties of bean (such as red kidney, black and cannellini beans). Add a handful of chopped fresh herbs, such as parsley, lots of spring onion, maybe some diced tomatoes or cucumber, and a tangy dressing of 1tbsp of apple cider vinegar and 2tsp of olive oil, salt and pepper.

Fats

The final section of the wholesome half of your plate should be food containing healthy fat. Unsaturated fats are generally the healthier versions. These are fats such as those found in olive oil, avocados and walnuts, which support heart health and provide necessary nutrients. Polyunsaturated fats, particularly omega-3 fatty acids from sources like oily fish and flaxseed, play a crucial role in reducing inflammation and alleviating joint pain, which can be especially beneficial during menopause.

My top tip to add healthy fats into your day

- Stock up on mixed nuts, put them in glass jars and if possible, keep them visible at home to remember to snack on a handful of nuts each day. Professor Sarah Berry says, 'Nuts are so good for you, so include a handful every day if you can.'

- Sprinkle a tablespoon of walnuts or a teaspoon of flaxseeds over your morning porridge or yoghurt.
- Drizzle a tablespoon of raw extra virgin olive oil over your meals just before serving – it works on salads, soups and steamed vegetables.

I hope, having shown you what's on your menopause plate, that you feel better equipped to plan balanced, nutrient-dense meals that fully support your health and wellbeing and your menopausal self. With this approach, each mealtime becomes an opportunity to fuel your body with the right mix of nutrients. 'Next time you're enjoying a simple dish like avocado on toast, remember that a few easy additions like mackerel or a couple of eggs can elevate it from a snack to a complete, satisfying meal,' says Julie. 'And don't pin all your hopes on one food or one meal or even on one day. It's the bigger picture that will make a difference to how you feel.'

Let the principles behind this plate become your guide to making mindful dietary choices that help to support you and your body in the best way.

Guidelines on How to Eat After Cancer

While this chapter is all about how diet can help you manage menopause symptoms after cancer, I also know that, as a cancer survivor, you're most likely curious about the broader guidelines for nutrition and recovery. Even though you now know that a Mediterranean style of eating can help ease your menopause symptoms, you may still wonder if there are foods to avoid post-cancer diagnosis, or if there is a particular way to eat after cancer, or if any foods cause cancer. Years ago, when I asked my oncologist if changing my diet could help keep cancer at bay, I was told, 'Not really, just eat as normal.' Needless to say, I was really unhappy with that answer. I just couldn't believe diet didn't matter. I mean, isn't it obvious that eating fast food every day wouldn't have the same effect as a balanced, nutritious diet? That brush-off actually fuelled my determination to dig a little deeper to understand the role of food in recovery and prevention and to find out how nutrition could truly support my body in the long run. The clearest guidance I found is provided by the American Institute for Cancer Research (AICR). They looked at the connection between diet, lifestyle, cancer, risk and survivorship in over 10,000 studies. Based on their research, and from their conclusions, their world-renowned independent researchers have developed the most reliable cancer prevention lifestyle advice currently available.[123] Most experts agree that cancer survivors should eat the same diet that is recommended to reduce cancer risk. This may help prevent a cancer from coming back or another type of cancer from occurring.

Here I have picked out the diet-specific points from AICR's cancer prevention guidance, available on their website.[124] Please refer to your digital handbook to download the full guidance.

1. Be a healthy weight. Keep your weight within the healthy range and avoid weight gain in adult life. The evidence linking obesity to cancer is overwhelming and has grown stronger over the past decade.

2. Eat a diet rich in whole grains, vegetables, fruits and beans. Make whole grains, vegetables, fruits and legumes such as beans and lentils a major part of your normal diet. A healthy pattern of eating

and drinking is associated with a lower risk of cancer. Independent studies show that the more closely you follow our recommendations, the more you reduce your risk of developing cancer.

3. Limit consumption of fast foods and other processed foods that are high in fat, starches or sugars. Limiting these products helps you control your calorie intake and makes it easier to maintain a healthy weight. There is strong evidence that diets containing greater amounts of fast foods and other processed foods high in fat, starches or sugars are a cause of weight gain, overweight and obesity. Greater body fatness is a cause of at least 12 cancers.

4. Limit consumption of red and processed meat. Eat no more than moderate amounts (12–18 ounces per week [340–510g]) of red meat, such as beef, pork and lamb. Eat little, if any, processed meat. There is strong evidence that eating red or processed meat are both causes of colorectal cancer.

5. Limit consumption of sugar-sweetened drinks. Drink mostly water and unsweetened drinks. There is strong evidence that regularly drinking sugar-sweetened drinks is a cause of weight gain, overweight and obesity.

6. Limit alcohol to reduce cancer risk. For cancer prevention, it is best not to drink alcohol. There is strong evidence that drinking alcohol is a cause of six cancers, and even one small glass of alcohol a day can increase the risk of some cancers.

For anyone who, like me, has ever wondered what to eat – or avoid – after a cancer diagnosis, I hope that sharing this guidance helps clarify some helpful steps you can take, one meal at a time. But just a word of encouragement: If your current diet feels far from the guidance offered here, it's normal to feel a bit of worry or even guilt about not getting everything 'right'. Maybe you eat processed meats a few times a week, or you drink alcohol regularly. As Julie said, let's keep blame and guilt out of the picture as you reflect on where you are right now. Should you want to make some dietary changes, you now know which direction to move in.

Most Frequently Asked Questions

At the workshops we host, certain questions come up frequently, so I wanted to address them here.

Does sugar feed cancer?

When I asked, 'Does sugar feed cancer?' during a podcast interview with Hillary Wright, a registered and licensed dietitian based in the US with over thirty years of experience, she shared that it's one of the most common concerns she hears from patients. Hillary is also the co-author of *The Menopause Diet Plan*, a book I can highly recommend. She explains: 'The idea that "sugar feeds cancer" is a common myth that oversimplifies a more complex relationship between cancer cells and glucose. It implies that eating something sugary, like a piece of chocolate cake, will immediately and directly fuel cancer cells. In reality, all cells in the body, both healthy and cancerous, use glucose as fuel. Eating sugar doesn't uniquely target cancer cells; rather, it raises blood-sugar and insulin levels, which all cells use for energy. While cancer cells do use more glucose due to their rapid growth, cutting out sugar alone doesn't "starve" cancer cells without also affecting healthy cells. Even if you significantly reduce sugar in your diet, your body has clever mechanisms (like breaking down carbohydrates, proteins and even fats) to maintain blood-glucose levels. Therefore, it's nearly impossible to deprive cells of glucose just by cutting out dietary sugar.'

'The problem arises with people regularly consuming high-sugar foods as part of their normal diet, as this leads to frequent blood-sugar spikes, which in return increase insulin production and, with time, insulin resistance. It is this constant insulin exposure that can contribute to an environment that encourages cell proliferation, potentially impacting cancer risk and other chronic health issues.'

How does sugar impact menopause symptoms?

Most of us know that it is healthy to limit excessive added sugar for our overall health. But what does regularly consuming sugar do to our menopause symptoms? 'Well, it can certainly make some of your symptoms worse,' explains nutritional therapist Julie Webb. 'When oestrogen drops due to cancer treatment and the onset of menopause, we become less insulin sensitive and may respond to carbohydrates less favourably. When we eat large amounts of carbohydrates, especially refined carbohydrates or sugars, such as white bread and baked goods, white rice and pasta, sugary snacks and drinks, they break down quickly into glucose, leading to a large and possibly rapid increase in blood-sugar levels. This "blood-sugar spike" triggers the release of insulin to help cells absorb glucose and bring blood-sugar levels back down to normal. This is a completely natural process and nothing to worry about. The issue arises with high glucose spikes and drops. This can lead to quick energy highs and then energy lows, causing irritability, anxiety, and fatigue.'

We know that the lack of oestrogen during menopause impacts mood, fatigue and anxiety, so these additional blood-sugar swings can make mood shifts feel even more intense. Additionally, when blood-sugar rises sharply, the body releases excess insulin to bring it down. If levels drop too quickly, it triggers the release of stress hormones like cortisol and adrenaline. This in return, can increase feelings of anxiety and exacerbate mood swings. Consistently high blood-sugar and insulin levels can also interfere with serotonin production. This neurotransmitter is also responsible for helping regulate mood, and lower serotonin levels can lead to symptoms like depression and irritability, which are already common during menopause.

Julie goes on, 'A drop in blood sugar can wake you up in the middle of the night. When blood-sugar levels dip too low, the body releases stress hormones to raise glucose levels, which can disrupt your sleep. So yes, it is fair to say, a diet high in sugar can make your menopause symptoms worse. It's best to have any of your sugary foods either in the day or straight after dinner, and well before bedtime to avoid a possible waking in the night. This is why I am so passionate that people look at their plates and try to include the nourishing half and the wholesome half of foods into each of their meals. It is the balance and combination of foods in one meal that will help prevent excessive spikes and drops in blood-sugar levels, which in return can help stabilise mood, reduce night-time wakings and improve overall energy levels.'

Hillary Wright adds that physical activity can help regulate blood-sugar and insulin levels, making it a powerful strategy for both cancer prevention and survivorship. Moving around for a bit or going for a walk after you eat can reduce your blood-sugar spikes.

Are phytoestrogens safe to eat?

Many people, especially those with a history of hormone-sensitive cancer, think they should avoid phytoestrogens in foods at all costs. Your doctor may have told you, 'You can't have oestrogen,' and now you think you need to avoid phytoestrogens in foods too. This is such a common question – I don't think we've ever hosted a workshop on diet where it didn't come up – so let's look at it in detail. 'You do not need to avoid eating phytoestrogens, this is another myth,' says Hillary Wright, and Julie adds, 'When I tell my clients their fears are not warranted, I am usually met with either relief or scepticism.' Phytoestrogens are plant compounds found in various foods, particularly soy products, flaxseeds, sesame seeds, whole grains and legumes, and including them in your diet can bring with it a number of health benefits. In the book *The Complete Guide to POI and Early Menopause,*[125] the authors write, 'Although their chemical structure is similar to oestrogen, *they are not the same as oestrogen*, and there is *no need to avoid these foods* even if you have been diagnosed with an oestrogen-dependant disease or condition.'[126]

There are two major classes of phytoestrogens: isoflavones and lignans. Isoflavones are the most common form, with the greatest dietary source being soya (edamame beans, tofu, tempeh, soy milk, miso). Other legumes, such as chickpeas and green peas, also contain isoflavones but in significantly lower levels. The second most-abundant class of phytoestrogen, lignans, is mainly present in flaxseed, although whole grains, vegetables and tea are also sources. Because of their oestrogenic effects in the body, phytoestrogens can be helpful in supporting menopausal symptoms. Research shows that including them in a balanced, whole-grain, plant-focused diet has health benefits from reducing hot flushes to improving bone health.

Some women who take tamoxifen have additional worries around phytoestrogens such as flaxseed, but current evidence suggests that flaxseed is safe for people who are on tamoxifen.[127] Not only are they safe but, like soya, flaxseed may in fact be beneficial to those with breast cancer and who are on tamoxifen; studies suggest that its consumption may reduce the risk, growth and recurrence of breast cancer. However, more clinical studies are needed to confirm this. Current recommendations advise those with hormone-sensitive cancers not to include phytoestrogen in supplement form, as long-term research is lacking – for more information about this, please see pages 169–171.

Can soy help with menopause symptoms?

You may be wondering if soy consumption can help ease menopause symptoms, as there is certainly a lot of talk about it everywhere you look. I wanted to understand the latest research into soy and consulted Professor Sarah Berry of King's College London and ZOE for help. In our deep dive on soy, Professor Berry explained, 'There are hundreds and hundreds of studies published looking at supplementing people with all sorts of things. The results are really inconsistent. I don't believe any single food or nutrient is universally effective in easing menopause symptoms. However, one exception is soy isoflavones, a type of phytoestrogen with a chemical structure similar to oestrogen. In regions with high soy consumption, like East Asia, some menopausal symptoms, like hot flushes for example, tend to be less common than in areas with low soy intake, such as the UK and the US.

Soy isoflavones contain different chemical compounds with varying potency. Evidence suggests a dose of above 15 milligrams of dioxin, which is one particular part of soy isoflavones as a supplement, has indeed a positive effect on significantly reducing menopause symptoms. However, this isn't the same for everyone, and it is this nuance that I am so passionate about explaining. Soy isoflavones affect different people differently, depending on their unique microbiome. As research into the microbiome and menopause continues to evolve, we are learning more about how our bodies interact with food and how tailoring our nutrition can help us feel our best. For me, understanding these nuances has reinforced that, until we know more, no single food or one meal will make a huge difference. Instead, I focus on incorporating a wide variety of foods into my meals, including soy, as and when it feels right for me.

A word of caution: as we have already seen, the supplement market is unregulated, and soy isoflavones in supplement form are currently contraindicated for some people with hormone-sensitive cancers as long-term research is lacking. If in doubt, don't use soy supplements, but feel free to include soy foods in your balanced meals and enjoy them as part of your varied diet.

Can I have meat if I have or have had cancer?

There is so much confusion and I hear so many questions around meat. There are many links between red and processed meat and cancer, probably the most well-known one being that processed meats or having a diet high in red meat are a cause of bowel cancer. These meats can also be high in calories and fat, which can contribute to weight gain.

While there are downsides to red and processed meat, the WCRF acknowledges that it can still be a good source of protein, iron, vitamin B12 and zinc, which can be beneficial for those who have cancer or have had cancer. There is no evidence to suggest you should avoid meat altogether.

Red meat includes beef, pork, mutton, lamb and goat. Chicken, turkey or other poultry count as white meat. White meat is lower in calories and saturated fat. Processed meat includes bacon, sausages, salami, chorizo, corned beef, hot dogs and all types of ham.

If you eat meat, eat a maximum of three portions of red meat a week. This is 525–750g of raw (equivalent to 350–500g of cooked) red meat per week. A portion of meat should fit into the size of your palm. If you do eat red meat, cutting down can help protect against bowel cancer.

Eat very little, if any, processed meat; there is strong evidence to show that it can be high in fat and salt, and eating it is a cause of bowel cancer. 'I advise all of my clients to start by just noting how much red or processed meat they consume each week, if any,' says Julie. 'You can then start planning how to go about reducing your meat intake should you wish to. In many cases, you may only need to make a few tweaks to reach the recommendations as in the guidelines.'

Does eating meat negatively impact menopause symptoms?

Eating red meat within the recommended guidelines is unlikely to make menopause symptoms worse for most individuals. While red meat and other animal products have long been linked to increased inflammation – which could potentially worsen symptoms like joint pain or hot flushes – research shows that this is typically only the case when red and/or processed meat is consumed excessively and as part of a diet high in ultra-processed foods.[128]

As outlined in this chapter, you're most likely to reduce your menopause symptoms by adopting a Mediterranean-style approach to eating. Julie Webb always emphasises not pinning all your hopes on the exclusion or inclusion of any single food group the same goes for red meat.

One thing I have learned over the years while hosting the SuperFood SupperClubs and speaking to so many survivors about diet is that if you want to reduce your red meat intake, for example, you have to plan what to replace it with. Make sure your alternatives are protein-rich and minimally processed. One common mistake I've seen people make when reducing meat is substituting it with highly processed vegan options, which often provide little nutritional benefit.

How much alcohol is safe to drink?

Consuming alcoholic drinks increases the risk of at least seven different types of cancer.[129] Alcohol, alongside asbestos, tobacco, radiation and processed meats, has been classed as a group 1 carcinogen by the International Agency for Research on Cancer (IARC), meaning there is no safe level of alcoholic drink consumption for cancer prevention. I know this is a tough one to read for many. Since there is no safe amount of alcohol, we know that the more you drink alcohol, the higher your risk of cancer. Conversely, the less you drink, the lower your cancer risk. Remember, it does not mean that if you drink alcohol it will give you cancer – but it will increase your risks of cancer. In a society where drinking alcohol is as socially accepted and expected as lighting a candle on a birthday cake, this message undoubtedly will come with mixed feelings for many of you. Feelings of guilt – 'Did my drinking cause cancer', to 'I know I really should stop drinking, but it's so hard. It feels like such a challenge, and I know I'll miss it more than I'd like to admit'. – are very normal and common.

Years ago, when I changed my diet overnight, I also stopped drinking alcohol. It was 1 January 2014 and it felt easiest to say to people that I was doing 'dry January'. For me, January rolled into February and into the rest of the year and, today, I still am not drinking any alcohol. Back then, I had no idea of any of the stats around alcohol and cancer risk, I just wanted to do everything possible to look after myself as best as I could. Besides, my hangovers post chemotherapy became awful and I did not want to waste any of my precious days on not feeling as good as I could. The first few months were the hardest. I had to justify myself at dinner parties and some friends felt let down that I was not joining in the drinking at birthdays; it really changed a lot about me and my social life and my connections to people. Not drinking alcohol had a massive impact on my life. And although it was tough for the first year, it also came with one of the most profound positive changes alongside my other newly found lifestyle habits. Being sober all the time means always being 'me' – showing up as who I really am, meeting my feelings and emotions all the time. I had to learn new strategies to relax, wind down and 'let go'. All this has come with so many powerful transformations.

For me, I also knew quitting alcohol was a better solution than just drinking less. I had tried that before, but because I was constantly having conversations in my own head about 'when to drink', 'how much to drink' and 'what to drink' it became tough work and all-consuming. The simpler option, for me personally, was not to drink at all.

Now, I know you will be faced with your own thoughts about what to do, and quitting alcohol may not be possible for some of you right now. One thing that is key to remember is that no one thing alone is ever going to give us cancer. Getting cancer is really bad luck. Some things, like alcohol, can increase our risks, but that's all. And just like with all the other strategies in the book: remember you don't have to do it all by yourself. There is help out there should you want to cut down on your alcohol intake. You can find alcoholic addiction support services in your local area by doing a quick search online. If you'd like to hear a non-judgemental enquiry into what happened when I gave up alcohol, I've linked a solo podcast episode for you in your digital handbook.

Does alcohol make your menopause symptoms worse?

Nutritional therapist Julie Webb explains: 'When it comes to the impact alcohol has on menopause symptoms, you may have already experienced the connection. There's no doubt about it: alcohol increases the likelihood of your hot flushes and night sweats. This in turn may then decrease the quality of sleep, causing fatigue, brain fog and anxiety the following day. The trouble is, for most people alcohol feels good in the moment – but the knock-on effect is rarely a positive one. Start by noticing how and if alcohol impacts your menopause symptoms over the next few weeks. Has the impact of a glass of wine changed since your cancer diagnosis and onset of menopause, or is it the same as before? Do you notice any changes to your sleep, hot flushes and other symptoms? Once you understand how alcohol impacts you, you can decide if you want to make changes to your drinking and if the benefits will be worth it for you.'

Can I drink coffee?

Caffeine found in coffee, green and black tea is often linked to increased menopause symptoms. Caffeine can stimulate the central nervous system, increasing heart rate and metabolism, which may make hot flushes and night sweats more intense. It can also increase anxiety and sleep disturbances. However, Julie says, 'But coffee and tea are also high in polyphenols (and pleasure!). Therefore, I'd say include them in your diet if you enjoy them. Decaffeinated tea and coffee are just as high in polyphenols. However, it is worth pointing out a few caveats. Since we know that caffeine can promote hot flushes and night sweats for some people, as indeed can all hot drinks and spicy foods, it might be worth cutting down or even cutting out caffeine to see if this helps. Make it an experiment and see if you notice any difference. It's also important to note that some people are fast metabolisers of caffeine, and this might promote feelings of anxiety and heart palpitations as the caffeine becomes available quickly. You may need to space your caffeinated drinks out or consume smaller drink sizes. And if you're a slow metaboliser of caffeine, you might need to be mindful of how late in the day you have your last caffeinated drink. After twelve hours, half the caffeine can still be in your system, which in turn may impact your sleep. Be your own detective here!'

What's the link between gut health and menopause symptoms?

There is so much talk about gut health, but I wondered if it was linked to menopause. Professor Sarah Berry explained to me that, 'There's interesting evidence to show that there's a relationship between the microbiome and menopause symptoms.[130 131] Just to clarify: the trillions of bacteria, fungi, protozoa and other microbes in your digestive tract make up your gut microbiome. The composition of that microbiome is unique to you. It influences your body's responses to food and is important for your overall health. The fact that there is a relationship between what you eat, your microbiome and many metabolic diseases is well known. In fact, having a thriving, varied gut microbiome is important for overall health – not just gut health. The more diverse a gut microbiome the better.

We now have some data to show that the microbiome composition is different depending on whether you're pre- or postmenopausal. This is because sex hormones affect your gut bacteria and, when hormone levels have changed with menopause, it makes sense that there are changes in your gut microbiome as well. Higher levels of oestrogen and progesterone levels boost gut bacteria diversity by feeding them. In some studies, we found a decrease in gut bacteria diversity after menopause or in women with low oestrogen levels. We also found that blood sugar, blood fat and inflammation markers were higher in postmenopausal women than those who hadn't yet gone through menopause. Changes in the microbiome also suggest that the way your body metabolises fat can change as a result of menopause, contributing to changes in weight. We need to carry out much, much more research into menopause to fully understand what that means for women's health. But the good news is that you can modify and improve your microbiome through dietary changes. What you eat matters!'

Sarah has some top tips for good gut health:

- Adopt the Mediterranean-style diet and remember food variety is key. Aim for 30 different plants (herbs and spices count too!) each week. Try to 'eat the rainbow' by eating plant foods in a mix of different colours.

- Eat more fruit and vegetables; many plants contain polyphenols and we know they have a range of health benefits for you.

- Add nuts and seeds; they contain healthy fats, such as omega-3 fatty acids, which are linked to a more diverse gut microbiome.

- Add legumes (lentils, chickpeas, soybeans, peas) and beans to your diet and make them part of your regular meals.

- Eat more whole grains (oats, quinoa, spelt, buckwheat); they too are associated with better gut health.

- Eat prebiotic foods; these nourish your 'good' gut bacteria. They are found in fruits such as blueberries and bananas, and cereals such as oats and rye, as well as nuts, onions and garlic.

- Eat probiotic foods; These contain live bacteria that may help increase the diversity of your gut bacteria. Anything fermented is great: sourdough bread, natural yoghurt, kefir, kombucha, pickles, miso, kimchi, tempeh.

- Avoid ultra-processed foods and cut down on sweets and cakes.

- Get good sleep, move regularly and lower your stress levels if you can, as this too will have an impact on your gut health.

My top tip to boost your gut health

- Make yourself a daily snack bowl using a minimum of six whole foods. It's a super-easy way to add a variety of foods without worrying about what recipe to follow. Mix fruit and veggies with cheese and tangy foods, such as olives, kimchi, some oatcakes – just make it a minimum of six, and mix it up every day. The more variety the better!

REFLECTIONS

Take a few moments to reflect...

1. Did you know the guidelines on diet for cancer survivors existed? And do you find it helpful knowing what they are?
2. How far off are you from the current guidance on nutrition for cancer survivors?
3. Reflect on how food makes you feel. Is there some guilt wrapped up in it, or feelings of 'not trying hard enough'?

POSITIVE ACTIONS

1. Keep a food diary and jot down everything you are consuming for a few days. Be honest!
2. Don't judge, or compare yourself to others – start by mapping out a simple plan for improving how you eat. Take some time to write a shopping list – it's a good starting point.
3. Plan *how* you are going to do it, don't just focus on what you want to do. It's often not enough. Fail to plan = Plan to fail.
4. Enjoy and celebrate your meals and eat consciously.
5. Use the symptom checker to keep track of your symptoms and see if your changes to your eating habits are helping you feel better.

CHAPTER 11
SYMPTOM TROUBLESHOOTER

Having facilitated numerous workshops and shared countless moments of walking, talking, laughing and crying with our community, I understand that sometimes you just want straightforward advice on how to manage a specific symptom.

We often receive messages on our community page like, 'I struggle to hold my pee despite doing pelvic floor exercises. Do I have to wear pads for the rest of my life, or is there anything that can help?'

A flurry of supportive messages usually follows, showcasing our incredible community spirit. This, alongside top tips and advice from doctors shared with me on podcasts and during interviews as part of my research for this book, is what I want to convey in this chapter. Many of the recommendations are backed by randomised control trials and some are based on anecdotal evidence. This way, you can see what others have found helpful and what doctors might recommend and decide what might work best for you.

Please refer back to the previous chapters to understand how some of the strategies mentioned here work. I go into more detail in those sections, but my aim for this chapter is to give you an at-a-glance summary of how you can begin tackling some of your most bothersome menopause symptoms.

Anxiety

Anxiety is a symptom of the menopause, but it can be amplified for cancer survivors due to both the physical stress of treatment and the psychological impact of navigating a serious illness. 'Anxiety presents differently for everyone,' explains Dr Nina Fuller-Shavel, an integrative medicine doctor specialising in integrative cancer support encompassing both mental and physical symptoms. 'While some people may only associate anxiety with worry, it can also manifest as irritability, difficulty concentrating or restlessness, or you may have specific fears, like scan-related anxiety or fear of recurrence. Physical symptoms are equally important and may include chest tightness, shortness of breath, heart palpitations, stomach discomfort, nausea, headaches, trouble sleeping and increased fatigue.'

In all the years of having navigated cancer survivorship and then early menopause, this has been a constant symptom and the most debilitating one for me. I wish that in the early years after treatment, I had gone and sought more help. Looking back, I thought feeling anxious after cancer was just part of the process. But it was more than that – it was draining, affecting my mental health, and holding me back from fully embracing life. The weight of constant worry became overwhelming at times. 'It is really important to know that whatever diagnosis you have, whatever stage you're at, whatever treatment you're going through, you do not need to suffer with mental health-related symptoms on top of your treatment and think that there is nothing you can do,' adds Dr Fuller-Shavel.

If you're unsure where to start, you can use the generalised anxiety disorder questionnaire (GAD-7), an online screening tool consisting of seven questions, which can help you assess your anxiety levels. This might help you to seek appropriate support from healthcare providers if needed. It's not a self-diagnosis, but it can be a first step before you seek support. Sometimes it's helpful to be able to use a tool like this to be able to say, 'Yes, my symptoms actually really do warrant help.' Personally, I think going through the questionnaire would have given me the confidence to take the next step to seek professional help.

Options and solutions

- Dr Fuller-Shavel explains that anxiety is a normal defence mechanism in our bodies. Our nervous system is saying, 'I'm worried about something. Something might be a threat.' She suggests that it's helpful to take a minute and acknowledge any bodily sensations or thoughts and recognise them as anxiety. This disempowers anxiety a little bit because we've taken the time to name it and acknowledge it rather than push it away.

- The UK's NICE guidelines[132] suggest starting to address anxiety using interventions such as cognitive behavioural therapy (CBT).

- Dr Fuller-Shavel explains, 'CBT is the primary treatment for anxiety for cancer survivors, but don't assume you're a hopeless case if CBT or talking therapy hasn't worked for you.'

- Additionally, the American Society for Clinical Oncology (ASCO) provides the following evidence-based recommendations on integrative approaches to managing anxiety and depression symptoms in adults living with cancer: mindfulness-based interventions (MBIs), yoga, acupuncture, tai chi and/or qigong, and reflexology for treating anxiety symptoms after cancer treatment.[133]

- Medication can also be considered – the first-line treatment after psychological therapy is usually sertraline, an SSRI (selective serotonin reuptake inhibitor). If SSRIs are ineffective, the next step is SNRIs (serotonin and noradrenaline reuptake inhibitors).

- Third-line options include medications, such as pregabalin. It's important to discuss the potential side effects and risks of these medications with your prescriber, as they can sometimes initially worsen symptoms before providing relief. Careful consideration and professional guidance are crucial when choosing the right medication.

- Beta-blockers are another form of medication used, primarily for symptomatic relief of anxiety, especially for palpitations or migraines. They work by blocking the effect of adrenaline on its receptor.

What I have been learning from the women in our community, however, is that lots of people use different, and often multiple, strategies to help ease their anxiety. For me this makes the most sense. When dealing with anxiety, there is likely not to be a one-size-fits-all approach and it's undoubtedly more effective to adopt a pick 'n' mix strategy. Women have told me that they have used all and any of the following, in combination, to address anxiety:

1. Exercise

2. Less alcohol

3. Daily walks

4. Share openly with friends and family

5. Antidepressants

6. CBT (see pages 191 – 195)

7. Counselling and talking therapy (see pages 200–202)

8. A gratitude journal (see pages 212–214)

9. Calming breaths and meditation

10. Yoga (see pages 205–208)

11. Cold showers

12. Let yourself cry

The main issue with some of this, however, is access; many of these strategies come with a financial cost that will be too much for many.

We have looked at, for example, online yoga classes that can be accessed through charities and teachers who provide free classes (including Vicky Fox, who we've already heard from).

You can try to access CBT through your doctor on the NHS. Additionally, look back at the Complementary Therapies chapter to explore how you can access CBT through online programmes.

The solution, in my opinion, is to acknowledge that your anxiety is real and that although it's common among cancer survivors, it does not mean you have to suffer it alone. Start somewhere. Reach out to your doctor and ask what they can do for you. Get the ball rolling and at the same time contact a local charity and ask what services and classes they provide. Doing something will always feel better than doing nothing.

Brain Fog

'Brain fog, though not a medical term, is a common way to describe a state of cognitive confusion such as forgetfulness, feeling less sharp, fuzzy-headed, difficulty concentrating, trouble finding words, and losing track of items or appointments,' explains dietician Barbie Boules. A similar term, 'chemo brain', is used to describe cognitive changes that some people experience during or after cancer treatment, also known as cancer-related cognitive impairment. It has symptoms similar to brain fog, which also negatively affect daily functioning and quality of life.

So many people I know say that brain fog is one of their most troublesome symptoms, resulting in them having to reduce their hours at work or even having to give up work altogether. The loss of confidence that comes with brain fog is real. For some, it is so life-impacting that they consider pausing or stopping their endocrine treatment in the hope of finding some normality. 'I wish there was such a thing as brain lube,' says Helen Addis, a breast cancer survivor and campaigner who was struggling on tamoxifen. Many people find it really hard to know what's what – is it brain fog caused by the menopause or is it chemo brain? Or maybe it's both? Some women I speak to worry that it might even be the onset of dementia.

Although it can be easy to think it's all to do with declining oestrogen levels, Barbie Boules explains, 'Brain fog can be caused by various factors such as stress, anxiety, depression, hormonal changes, poor sleep quality, diet and even certain medications.' Dr Lindsey Thomas, an experienced GP and menopause specialist who sees cancer patients as part of her NHS work, echoes this: 'Often, it's impossible to say whether it is the chemotherapy causing the brain fog or whether it is the lack of hormones, because there's such a mix of things going on there. Usually when I see cancer patients other symptoms are going on alongside the brain fog, so women who are struggling with their menopause might not be sleeping well, their stress levels might be higher and they might be feeling more anxious. They might be exhausted and relying on options that can give a quick fix, such as food choices, caffeine and perhaps alcohol. But ultimately all of these can make brain fog worse.'

Options and solutions

Boules explains that to address brain fog it can be helpful to act a bit like a detective to establish what's going on. Sometimes small adjustments like improving sleep quality, reducing alcohol or caffeine intake and drinking more water can significantly alleviate symptoms.

Most experts will agree that combating brain fog requires a multitude of strategies. Adequate oestrogen levels, if possible, are a great starting point. For those for whom hormone therapy is not advised, though, it's important to look at working towards a multifaceted approach:

- Sleep quality is a good start (see pages 304–308).
- Ensure you're hydrated well – many people just don't drink enough water!
- Monotask: Close down all the many tabs on your computer, leave your phone in a different room when you complete tasks so that you don't get too distracted.
- Write lists and set alarms on your phone to remind you of important things.

- Nutrition is key, so make sure your intake of omega-3s (DHA and EPA), B12, vitamin D and choline is sufficient to support cognitive function.

- Balance meals to stabilise blood sugars (see pages 247–256).

- Regular exercise, especially in the morning, enhances circulation and concentration throughout the day.

- Take yourself for regular walks, even short ones. People who do brisk walking every day have much better cognitive function than people who don't do anything at all.

- Plan ahead for the cringeworthy moments when you can absolutely not remember what you were saying halfway through a sentence. Put together a 'what will I say if...?' strategy. Sure, you can make a joke about it. Or you say, 'Gosh, I have gone blank – help me out here, where was I?' In most situations, people will be happy to help you get back on track. By being prepared you might go into situations feeling less anxious to begin with.

- Communicate openly: If you feel you can be open about what you are experiencing with your employers and people you work with, it can help take the pressure off at times when you don't feel quite as sharp or as quick as you used to be.

- Consider opening up and saying, 'Oh my goodness, my brain isn't working quite as I want it to today.'

Fatigue/Lack of Energy

Fatigue is not the same as being tired after a busy day or having an afternoon slump. Fatigue can impact you daily, mentally and/or physically, and it limits you in your daily activities. You just don't feel rested after sleeping. Tiredness, lack of energy and fatigue are symptoms so many of the women I speak to struggle with, yet it's hard to unpick why this is happening. Cancer treatments can take their toll and can cause fatigue. In many cases, regaining the energy you once had takes longer than you might expect. And menopause in its own right can cause fatigue too. Oestrogen and testosterone directly boost physical energy and drive, so of course if you are in a hormone-deficient state this will impact you greatly. We also know that 70–80 per cent of cancer survivors struggle with sleep, so, if you are not sleeping well, this too will add to you feeling fatigued during the day. Additionally, chronic stress can impact our energy levels and can be the cause of fatigue. For me, one of the hardest lessons, but one of the most impactful strategies for managing fatigue, was learning to say 'no' more often. By setting these boundaries, I was able to reclaim both time and energy, allowing me to focus on the things that truly mattered to me. It helped me avoid the exhaustion that comes from overcommitting but also gave me the space to fully engage in activities that brought genuine joy and fulfilment.

Options and solutions

- Firstly, if you are feeling tired all the time, speak to your doctor and ask for a full blood count. Ask to have your iron/ferritin levels checked, alongside your vitamin D, vitamin B12, folate levels, thyroid, liver and kidney function, as well as your inflammatory and diabetes markers. We often don't think about getting our basic blood levels taken, but this can be a helpful starting point to rule out any underlying deficiency or condition that needs treating.

- If you take HRT, then you can discuss with your doctor to be tested to make sure you are absorbing it correctly. Dr Hannah Short, co-author of *The Complete Guide to POI and Early Menopause,* told me about her own surgical-onset menopause and how hard it was for her to find the right hormone treatment due to absorption issues.

- Drink plenty of water.

- Make time for a short rest every day if you can. Plug yourself into a 15-minute guided meditation (free on our YouTube channel). Close your eyes and let your nervous system recharge. It's a non-negotiable for me.

- The Royal College of Occupational Therapists explains that 'The 3P strategy' can help you find ways to conserve your energy: Planning, Pacing, and Prioritising.[134] This common strategy is used to manage and combat fatigue, particularly for individuals with chronic illnesses or conditions that cause persistent tiredness. Here's a brief explanation of each:

    1. Planning: Organise your activities in advance to avoid overexertion. This involves scheduling tasks and allowing sufficient time for rest.

    2. Pacing: Balance activities with rest periods to prevent exhaustion. It's about doing activities at a steady pace rather than rushing.

3. Prioritising: Determine which tasks are most important and focus your energy on those, while possibly delegating or postponing less critical activities.

- Exercise might be the last thing you feel like doing, but we know that any movement, however small, can help our energy levels (see pages 220–222).

Genito-urinary Syndrome of Menopause (GSM)

This relatively new term presents a variety of symptoms, which can be broken down into three main areas: vulval, vaginal and bladder/urinary tract symptoms. Each set of symptoms relates to the loss of oestrogen, which affects the health and function of the genital and urinary areas. The symptoms of genito-urinary syndrome of menopause (GSM) include vulval dryness, itching, burning and increased sensitivity, which can cause discomfort during activities like sitting or sex. Vaginal symptoms, such as dryness, painful intercourse and reduced elasticity, often result in discomfort, pain or changes in discharge. Bladder and urinary symptoms, including frequent UTIs, urgency, incontinence and burning during urination, are common due to thinning tissues and reduced moisture. Despite over 80 per cent of women experiencing vaginal dryness, many find it difficult to discuss these issues with their doctors. We also know many doctors never ask about these symptoms as treatment side effects. As a result, many women suffer in silence. For the full list of symptoms please refer back to our symptom checker on page 34.

Options and solutions

- Basic vulval and vaginal care: Maintaining a good intimate health routine can keep your vulva, vagina and bladder healthy. When washing the vagina/vulva, avoid anything that might scratch or irritate the skin, such as flannels. Only use water or a gentle emollient. Our experts often say, 'Your vagina is a self-cleaning oven and does not require any douching.'

- Avoid any products that contain irritating ingredients. Stay away from glycerine, glycols and parabens, dyes, glitter and perfume.

- According to a vulval dermatologist, black underwear contains a dye that can irritate some vulvas. If possible, wear white cotton undies if you're uncomfy, and no tight clothes.

- Some women use a sitz bath (a warm-water bath you sit in to relieve discomfort in your perineal region) and specially designed cushions to sit on if things are really bad.

- Moisturise your vulva and vagina using skin-safe products (see pages 80–83).

- Use a skin-safe lubricant for intimacy and sex (see pages 80–83).

- Use a local/vaginal/topical oestrogen (see pages 124–134).

- Look into specific probiotics that support the microbiome of your vagina.

- Keep a bladder diary. This involves tracking the time and amount of urination, fluid intake, urgency and any urinary leakage or discomfort over several days to help identify patterns and manage urinary issues. A bladder diary is a practical tool that supports better management of bladder-related issues.

- My colleague Esther at Menopause and Cancer says, 'Having a physical examination is a must if you're having issues, as conditions like lichen sclerosis can crop up in menopause and that is diagnosed by sight or biopsy. Examine yourself in the mirror once a month. If something feels off, take a close look and note any changes. If you're unsure about anything, don't hesitate to see your GP. And seek help from a women's health physio to help you tailor pelvic floor physiotherapy according to your needs. Combining a few different strategies might give you the best results, so keep an open mind and start trying things out – there's a lot you can do.'

Refer back to Chapter 5 for more information on non-hormonal options, and also to the vaginal oestrogen section in Chapter 6 for a more detailed discussion on all things related to your sexual health.

Hot Flushes/Night Sweats

Hot flushes and night sweats, also called vasomotor symptoms, are common and distressing for menopausal women.[135] They may be infrequent and mild, or could be persistent throughout the day and night and be debilitating. The sudden bursts of heat, sweating and chills can certainly disrupt daily life and sleep. Some women also experience cold flushes and, in many cases and both kinds of flush, they come with heart palpitations and dizziness, which can make the whole experience very uncomfortable.

In menopause, hormonal changes, especially the decrease in oestrogen, disrupt the body's temperature regulation. In post-cancer patients, these symptoms tend to be more acute and severe. Hot flushes and night sweats can adversely impact energy levels, sleep, cognition and mood, leading to reduced quality of life. Many women I speak with express frustration when they receive well-meaning advice for hot flushes, such as 'bring a fan' or 'wear layers'. While these suggestions may offer some relief, they often don't make a significant enough difference for many people dealing with the intensity of these symptoms.

Options and solutions

- When hormone replacement therapy (HRT) is an option, it can be highly effective in managing hot flushes, providing significant relief from the frequency and intensity for many individuals.

- If HRT is contraindicated, there are other strategies and treatments. Some people really don't want any more medication and want to try a complementary therapy, for example, while others try combining a few different strategies in the hope of getting the most relief.

- Non-hormonal prescribable medications can provide relief from hot flushes. These are treatments your doctor can prescribe for you. For much more detailed information on all these prescribable non-hormonal treatment options, refer to Chapter 5.

- Complementary therapies such as acupuncture, visualisation and hypnosis can help; refer to Chapter 8.

- Avoiding triggers is a simple strategy you can apply that can make a significant difference. Common triggers for hot flushes include alcohol, caffeine, spicy foods and sugary foods. Some women also report that their hot flushes are worse after eating red meat. Additionally, taking hot baths or drinking hot beverages in the evening can lead to night sweats later in the night. Try to notice if, by adjusting any of these habits, you find better relief from your vasomotor symptoms.

- Staying hydrated is important, as dehydration can make hot flushes worse. Opt for water and herbal teas.

- For more information on how incorporating more plant-based foods, including switching to a high-fibre diet rich in phytoestrogens and soy, can help reduce the severity of your hot flushes, refer to Chapter 10.

- Wear comfortable clothing made from breathable fabrics, like cotton, bamboo or moisture-wicking materials. This can make a big difference as these fabrics help regulate your body temperature. Also, wear layers for temperature control.

- Invest in quality bedding if you can; breathable sheets made from cotton or linen can make you feel more comfortable in the night.

- Stress can cause hot flushes to worsen. Stress hormones like adrenaline can affect the body's temperature regulation, potentially increasing the frequency and intensity of hot flushes. By managing your stress you can help mitigate the severity of your hot flushes (see page 211 for guidance).

- Herbal medication can offer relief from hot flushes, especially for those unable to take hormone replacement therapy (HRT). Please see Chapter 8 for herbal medicine options; I also discuss how to go about choosing herbal supplements or how to work with a medical herbalist.

Infertility

Infertility induced by cancer treatment refers to the loss of the ability to conceive a child as a result of undergoing treatments for cancer. I am aware it's not a 'symptom' like the others I have listed here, but it's important to address. It can occur due to the effects of cancer therapies on the reproductive system. The degree of infertility depends on various factors, including the type and dosage of treatment and the age and reproductive health of the person before treatment. Even if you had not decided whether you wanted to become a biological mum, having that possibility taken away from you can feel devastating. Many people say that infertility is by far the hardest aspect of their cancer journey. Some of you reading this will have been able to embark on a type of fertility preservation, but for many people fertility preservation before cancer treatment is not possible for various reasons. Most likely, you have all been on a very challenging journey up until now. I am aware that I cannot do this sensitive subject justice by writing a small paragraph here in the book, but I also did not want to avoid addressing it. The psychological impact of infertility is undoubtedly very complex and personal and, while you may be dealing with a personal loss or the uncertainty of becoming a biological parent or not, you might also have to cope with others around you becoming parents. Helen Munro contacted me to share her story on the podcast. She had been diagnosed with breast cancer, and spoke so candidly about her loss of fertility after her diagnosis: 'It felt like everywhere I looked, people were pregnant. I felt so different and jealous, but more than jealous, it was much more complex than jealousy or envy. I was in this dark, dark place.' Helen went on to explain how she found a way through and how she eventually freed herself from the very dark place she was in.

Many other women also shared their stories with me. Most say how devastated they feel by losing their fertility to their cancer treatment. Since the emotional rollercoaster that accompanies fertility challenges can be overwhelming, a process of grief will most likely arise and it can take a long time, sometimes even a lifetime, to adapt. Like one lady wrote, 'Life looks very different this side of the diagnosis.' Kate Pleace, a fertility and menopause specialist nurse, has some practical advice:

- The first step in the fertility preservation journey is often the initial consultation with a fertility specialist. However, it is not uncommon for patients to feel overwhelmed during this appointment, as they are processing a cancer diagnosis and also navigating the complex world of fertility treatment. Often this is a time where everything feels rushed and, with hindsight, many people say they wish they had taken more time to absorb and understand the information given to them. Some cancer treatments will start immediately after diagnosis, but, if time allows, you and your doctors may decide to freeze your eggs or, if you are with a partner, your embryos, before you start your cancer treatment. At a later stage, thawed eggs can be fertilised with your partner's or a donor's sperm. Thawed embryos can also be replaced if they have survived the thawing process successfully. Another option is a newer and less common procedure called ovarian tissue preservation. It is a surgical procedure where a small amount of the ovary will be stored and frozen for future use. The goal is to have the option to replace it in the patient's body in future to potentially restart the cycles again.

- After taking the initial steps for fertility preservation, most individuals proceed with their cancer treatment, facing the dual challenge of managing both their cancer and the uncertainty surrounding their future fertility. This situation involves not only coping with the immediate effects and demands of cancer treatment but also grappling with the potential long-term impact on their ability to conceive. The process to explore the options around becoming a parent can continue at a later stage after cancer treatment. It will very much depend on the individual when and if the time is right. For some people periods might come back after treatment, for others they won't. For those in a relationship with a male partner, they might embark on using the frozen eggs at a later stage or to decide to thaw the embryos. For those without a male partner, donor sperm can be used to fertilise the eggs, which can create embryos that can be used as part of IVF treatment. Some women might want to consider embryo adoption, surrogacy or adoption; all are often complex emotional journeys for the intended parents.

- Regardless of where you are at in the process, the grief that comes with infertility and the uncertainty about your fertility is very real. It is not just about the loss of fertility, but the loss of a future and possibilities that you had imagined for yourself. Counselling can be incredibly supportive during the challenging time of cancer treatment and its impact on your ability to conceive, and I hope you have been able to access this type of help. Therapy, including grief counselling sessions, offers a safe space to navigate the emotional rollercoaster of facing potential infertility, helping you process feelings of loss, anxiety and uncertainty. It can also guide you through the transition to new realities, whether that means exploring alternative paths to parenthood or finding ways to cope with grief over changes in your life plans. Counselling can also help strengthen relationships with loved ones, as of course infertility will affect the whole family in different ways.

Joint Pains and Aches

Menopausal joint aches and pains, often referred to as arthralgia, can be common symptoms of menopause and may become more pronounced in women experiencing treatment-induced menopause after cancer therapy or for those on certain medications. Muscle pain and stiffness, sore joints or a body that's 'aching all over', restless legs, painful feet, pins and needles, frozen shoulder and carpal tunnel syndrome are all common menopause-related musculoskeletal symptoms.

So many of you tell me that you can hardly take your duvets off your bodies in the morning because your hands hurt, and that you hobble out of bed towards the bathroom in pain. 'I'm walking like a penguin,' say many. Our joints, muscles, ligaments and tendons are all depending on and interacting with sex hormones. Joint pain is a common symptom of the menopause and extremely common among cancer survivors, especially those on endocrine therapy.

The pain is most common in the hands and feet, but can also happen in the knees, hips, lower back and shoulders. You may have it all the time or it may come and go. You may notice that your joints are stiffer in the morning when you first get up. If you have recently started taking an aromatase inhibitor such as anastrozole, letrozole or exemestane, the pain may get better over the next few months. This may happen as the body adjusts to changes in hormone levels.

In a podcast episode with two menopause experts, Dr Melanie Hacking and Dr Susanne Hooper, I asked, 'What happens if we can't have oestrogen back and have really bad joint ache and joint pain?' Dr Hacking explained, 'While oestrogen plays a major part in joint health and there is no denying that, joint health is not just linked to oestrogen.'

Dr Hooper added, 'The key points are that joint pain during menopause has multiple causes. While oestrogen can help, a multimodal approach is necessary, including a low-inflammatory diet and regular movement.'

Options and solutions

- 'Lotion is Motion' and keep on moving is a key message most doctors will give you. And yet, it might be the last thing you want to do if you are in pain. You need to avoid your joints stiffening up even more because you're not using them, especially first thing in the morning. Before you even get out of bed, rotate your wrists and ankles, take some gentle stretches, and then get up. It can make all the difference. Gentle movement like yoga and Pilates is very helpful. One of the ladies in our community agrees: 'Sometimes it feels so counterintuitive to do the movement stuff when struggling with pain, but I honestly always feel better when I do it and definitely feel worse if I don't.'

- Getting some advice from a physio isn't a bad idea because not only can they recommend better movements for you, they can also suggest splints for wrists for example.

- Avoid processed foods as much as you can as this can increase inflammation. Inflammation in the body can make joint aches worse. As oestrogen levels drop, the body's ability to regulate inflammation may decrease, leading to more joint stiffness, swelling and discomfort. Oestrogen has an anti-inflammatory effect, so when its levels fall the joints can become more prone to inflammation, which can worsen pain and stiffness.

- Eating a lot of varied nutrients, not leaving out food groups and having a calcium-rich diet is important. Focus on a diet rich in magnesium-containing foods like nuts, seeds, leafy green vegetables and whole grains, or consider trying a magnesium supplement. Women say it helps with sleep, restless legs, joint aches and stiffness. Some studies suggest that if you have lower levels of vitamin D, taking vitamin D3 supplements may improve symptoms. Additionally, omega-3 is important for joint health, and you may want to consider a supplement. Glucosamine and chondroitin supplements are aimed at improving joint cartilage, which can be beneficial and safe, especially when combined with a varied diet. There is a lack of extensive evidence-based studies, which makes it hard for medical professionals to fully endorse these supplements, but they can be a good addition for those seeking extra joint support. Talk to your doctor before taking a supplement.

- There is some evidence supporting the benefits of collagen for joint health, but individual results can vary, with some saying they have not noticed any improvement. Refer to the herbal supplements section on pages 165–169 for more info.

- Controlling inflammation with medication can be helpful. Most people tolerate paracetamol well, and it can significantly improve symptoms, making it a useful option for managing pain. Though it doesn't cure the condition, it helps with symptom management. I've spoken to some ladies who manage their pain with paracetamol at weekends, when they want to be more active with their families.

- For those who prefer not to take tablets, there are topical treatments such as sprays, patches, gels and ointments. Topical non-steroidal anti-inflammatory drugs including ibuprofen can reduce inflammation and pain when applied directly to the affected joint. They can be a good option for targeting localised pain without the systemic effects. Menthol is a cooling agent that can provide temporary relief by stimulating nerve endings and creating a cooling sensation. Another option is capsaicin, which is derived from chilli peppers and is used in some topical ointments to block pain signals. However, if multiple joints are affected, using topical treatments all over may not be practical.

- Anti-inflammatories can be useful for managing pain, but they are harder to tolerate long term due to potential stomach issues. It's important to use them in moderation and with caution. Ibuprofen is part of the non-steroidal anti-inflammatory drugs family, which are commonly used to reduce mild to moderate inflammation and pain. Corticosteroids are more potent anti-inflammatories, often prescribed for more severe inflammation or chronic inflammatory conditions.

- Acupuncture can be a very useful treatment and help with symptom improvement of joint aches and pains.

- Hot and cold: The initial use of cold helps reduce inflammation, while heat applied afterwards promotes blood flow and healing. Opinions vary, with some preferring only heat and others only cold, including ice baths to limit inflammation. It's largely a matter of personal preference since there's no definitive evidence favouring one method over the other. The primary goal is to control inflammation, so you should use what feels best for you.

- You may have noticed that a certain brand of tamoxifen or other medication can make your joint ache worse. Take note of which brand you are being prescribed and see if it makes a difference to your symptoms.

- If the pain is difficult to cope with and you are on an aromatase inhibitor, for example, your cancer doctor may suggest changing the type of aromatase inhibitor you take. If that does not work, they may suggest you take tamoxifen instead. Tamoxifen causes fewer problems with joint pain. For more info go to Chapter 7 where I discuss in more detail how to navigate endocrine therapy.

- Members of our community have said that yoga, walking, magnesium sprays and balms, turmeric supplements, cold water immersions and Epsom salt baths help their achy joints and sore muscles.

Loss of Libido

A combination of factors can lead to a loss of libido, and it's more common than you may think. 'Anyone else struggling with low libido/ zero desire since menopause? My sex drive is non-existent and it's now having a major effect on my marriage, so if anyone's tried anything that's worked I'd be so grateful!', I hear so often. The emotional and psychological impact of cancer, including stress, anxiety and fear, can significantly reduce sexual desire. Cancer treatments such as chemotherapy, radiation and hormone therapies can have side effects like fatigue, pain and early menopause, which directly affect libido. Physical changes resulting from cancer or its treatments can also impact sexual function and body image, further diminishing interest in sex. And of course, the strain on relationships that comes with a life-changing diagnosis can contribute to a decreased libido. If you have a partner, they too will experience their own emotional and mental changes as they witness you going through treatment. Many people don't think there is much they can do about their loss of sex drive, hence most people don't ask for help. Of course, it's also quite embarrassing to talk about our sex lives.

All these factors (physical, psychological, emotional and interpersonal or societal) impact a person's experience of sexuality. When someone is diagnosed with cancer and undergoes treatment, each of these domains can be affected. Dr Angela Wright, a psychosexual therapist and menopause expert, with whom we have facilitated many workshops, offers some helpful advice:

Options and solutions

- 'If you're not enjoying sex as it hurts or because you don't get aroused, then of course libido falls because you're not getting a reward of any sort from it. You might even be getting something negative from it.' Dr Wright recommends washing, moisturising and massaging with a good emollient, using a skin-safe lube for any penetration, and in combination trying local vaginal and vulval oestrogens. For more detailed information on intimate care, moisturisers, lubes and vaginal oestrogen, see pages 80–83 and 124–134.

- But sexual health post-cancer isn't just about managing physical symptoms like vaginal dryness, though that's one part of it. Many patients avoid intimacy and many say, 'I am completely numb.' If you're in a relationship and you have stopped being intimate, this can lead to a significant change between you and your partner, where even simple acts like cuddling or going on a date night become rare. Some people feel worried the cuddling or kissing might lead to 'more' and they're not ready for that or have no desire to go there. Of course, when the cuddling stops, it can feel as if the gap between you and your partner becomes even greater. It can help simply to talk. For many couples, the conversation can feel hard to start, but communication is essential.

- Use 'I' statements, as these are less likely to provoke a defensive response. Explain how things are for you. Talk about what you fear. What you miss. Look for the shared ground. What did intimacy mean to one or both of you? What do you want more of? How can you find that? Sometimes it helps to agree on what you don't want to do for a while, in order to signal that other forms of intimacy are still welcome. Keep touching – especially non-intimate touch, as this helps build connection and permission for non-verbal expression between you.

- There can also be trauma from a cancer diagnosis, surgery or treatment, which can deeply affect our sense of safety and control over our bodies. Such trauma often arises from feeling unsafe or helpless and can leave our bodies feeling unfamiliar.

Unprocessed trauma may lead to emotional blocks or sudden, overwhelming feelings, making it difficult to stay present or communicate effectively. If you feel you have unprocessed trauma, it can be really helpful to find someone to talk to about this. Body-based methods like mindfulness, breath-based activities or yoga can be very effective in reconnecting with the body, and calming anxiety and trauma responses. These strategies can also help connect you back to your body.

- When it comes to sex, it can help a lot to explore things on your own first. What touch feels good now? Is there anything that feels uncomfortable? What sparks your interest, and what turns you off?

- Think about what you may need to feel relaxed, comfortable, and in the right space emotionally for sexuality. We often need to ensure that we are meeting most of our non-sexual needs before addressing our need for intimacy. This means rest, exercise, safety and having our emotional needs met. 'Getting back to sex can take time, so in the meantime agree to widen what counts as quality intimacy: sex is a buffet, not a three-course meal,' Dr Wright suggests.

- Try to get referred to a psychosexual therapist. They can help you work through the emotional impact of trauma and grief, support you in understanding and redefining your sexual identity and function, and improve how you communicate with your partner. They address specific issues like reduced libido or discomfort and teach you practical strategies and relaxation techniques to manage stress and boost intimacy.

- Some medications including antidepressants (gabapentin, oxybutynin), and those which help with sleep problems and hot flushes, can further reduce lubrication and libido, or delay climax. So basically, they can put the brakes on your sex drive. Do speak to your doctor if you are trying to improve your sex drive and are on any of these medications.

- Dr Wright explains that HRT, including testosterone, can be helpful for a loss of libido, and recommends it for women who are not contraindicated in taking it. She also explains that she increasingly uses medications called PDE5 inhibitors. These are drugs like Viagra, which can be used not just for men but also for women, especially those who can't or prefer not to use hormones. While these drugs are traditionally used to maintain blood flow to the genitals in men, they are showing promise in women as well. Dr Wright notes that this medication is used 'off-label'. Although this might sound worrying, off-label use is quite common, such as with certain birth control medication being used to treat acne, for example. While it may not be officially approved, it doesn't mean the medication is unsafe or unstudied. In women's health, where options can be limited, using medications creatively is often necessary.

- In addition, there are two drugs in the US, called Addyi (flibanserin) and Vyleesi (bremelanotide), that are approved for the treatment of hypoactive sexual desire disorder (HSDD), which is the condition of persistent or recurrent lack of sexual desire.

Osteoporosis/Osteopenia

Osteoporosis and osteopenia are both conditions related to bone density loss. Bone density refers to how thick and strong your bones are, and how likely they are to break. Osteopenia is an early stage of bone density loss, where bone mineral density (BMD) is lower than normal, and osteoporosis is a more advanced form, where bones become fragile, brittle and more prone to fractures, even with minor stress or injury. Chances are you worry about your bone health or you already know that your cancer treatment and menopause have impacted your bones in a negative way. The Royal Osteoporosis Society says one in two women over 50 in the UK will get a fracture due to osteoporosis. If you go through an early menopause – before 45 – or a premature menopause – before 40 – the situation is even worse and you are more likely to develop osteoporosis and have weaker bones in later life.[136] At every workshop, I bring up bone health, and I am often shocked when women tell me they had no idea their early menopause may impact their bone health in a negative way. But unless we know, we can't proactively do anything about it!

Several chemotherapy drugs can lead to reduced bone density, increasing the risk of osteoporosis and fractures. This is especially an issue with some breast cancer treatments, which suppress the production of the hormone oestrogen, the female hormone that maintains bone strength. With treatments such as Zoladex, which can temporarily suppress oestrogen production, studies have shown that women experience a loss of up to 5–10 per cent in bone density within two years. Aromatase inhibitors, too, increase the rate of bone loss and the risk of fractures. Tamoxifen is not associated with significant bone loss in postmenopausal women; the drug actually provides some bone protection. In contrast, tamoxifen can cause small decreases in bone density in premenopausal women in the first two years of treatment. A non-invasive DEXA scan (Dual-Energy X-ray Absorptiometry, see below and page 302) can measure your bone density, helping assess bone strength and the risk of fractures or osteoporosis.

GP and menopause expert Dr Olivia Hum, who I have had the pleasure of talking to at many workshops, offers some practical solutions for us below. She says, 'There are other factors that affect your risk of osteoporosis and mean that you may be at higher risk than other women taking the same treatment as you. These include lifestyle factors like smoking, having a high alcohol intake or leading a sedentary lifestyle. Having a low BMI (less than 19) or having an eating disorder puts you at higher risk. We also see more osteoporosis in women with some underlying medical conditions such as coeliac disease, rheumatoid arthritis and inflammatory bowel disease. It is also worth asking your mother whether she has ever had a diagnosis of osteoporosis or has had a hip fracture as this also significantly increases your own risk.'

Options and solutions

- If you have been through an early or premature menopause, or are worried about your bones, talk to your oncologist or your GP. They can help you assess your fracture risk and see whether you meet the criteria for having a DEXA scan. A DEXA scan is a medical imaging test used to measure bone density and assess bone health.

- Alternatively, if you have not had your bone health assessed by a healthcare professional, you can identify if you are at high risk for osteoporosis by taking the free online osteoporosis risk checker on the Royal Osteoporosis Society website.[137] This is based on the FRAX test, which is a tool that is used to evaluate the risk of fracturing a bone in the future.

- The Royal Osteoporosis Society advises that, if you have an early menopause, you should talk to your healthcare professional about whether you can take hormone replacement therapy (HRT) as this will be protective for your bones.[138] If you cannot take HRT due to the type of cancer that you have had, then there are other treatments available.

- If you are on treatments for breast cancer that can affect your oestrogen levels, and therefore bone strength, an assessment of your fracture risk should be made at some point in your treatment. Different centres have different protocols but it has been suggested that anyone who is under 45 and develops menopause caused by their treatment should have a DEXA scan. Many guidelines also suggest that postmenopausal women started on an aromatase inhibitors should also have a DEXA scan within three months of starting treatment. Ask your oncologist or breast care nurse what your local protocol says.

- After a DEXA scan you may be classified as at low, moderate or high risk of fracture. Women at high risk of fracture may be offered bisphosphonate medication.

- Bisphosphonates are medications that help prevent bone density loss by slowing down the cells that break down bone tissue. By inhibiting these cells, bisphosphonates help maintain or even increase bone density. These are either given as an oral tablet or as intravenous infusions. Some women experience gastrointestinal, joint and flu-like symptoms for a short period of time after taking the drugs.

- Sometimes, unfortunately, bone health can be forgotten about with the huge number of different things that have to be taken into account by your treating team when treating cancer. If you are taking one of the treatments mentioned above, or have undergone an early or premature menopause, you may sometimes have to remind your team that assessment of your fracture risk is an important part of your treatment.

- Building muscle is key to protect your bones. Not only do muscles hold up your skeleton, but having strong muscles reduces your risk of falling. Experts advise regularly engaging in weight-bearing and muscle-strengthening exercise.

- Ensure you take your vitamin D supplement. Public Health England advises adults and children over the age of one to take 10 micrograms (400 IU) of vitamin D each day to support bone and muscle health, as it can be hard to get enough from sunlight during the winter months in the UK.

- Load up on magnesium- and calcium-rich foods such as leafy green vegetables, nuts and seeds, fish, legumes, dairy and fortified non-dairy products. Check the Royal Osteoporosis Society calcium calculator to see how to get the recommended amount of calcium in your daily diet (more on page 182). It is not advised to take a calcium supplement unless you have been prescribed one. We know that healthy, balanced diets (high in fruit, vegetables, fish, poultry and whole grains) are beneficial for your bone strength.

- Stop smoking and keep alcohol to a minimum.

- The Strong, Steady, Straight Quick Guide by the Royal Osteoporosis Society is an excellent resource providing tips on exercises and lifestyle strategies to maintain strong bones, prevent falls and support good posture. Look it up![139]

- Refer to Chapter 10, and in particular pages 230–231, for the ins and outs of what exercise is best for bone health.

Poor Sleep/Insomnia

According to NICE guidelines, insomnia is difficulty in getting to sleep, early wakening or non-restorative sleep that occurs despite adequate opportunity for sleep. It is typically diagnosed when poor sleep occurs at least three times a week for three months or more, and it significantly affects daily functioning.

'For women in menopause after cancer, about 70–80 per cent of women describe poor sleep or insomnia, and many suffer for years after their active cancer treatment is completed,' says menopause doctor and sleep expert Dr Zoe Schaedel.

Many people in our community report trying everything to improve their sleep. They establish healthy sleep habits by creating a comfortable sleep environment and avoiding screens and heavy meals before bed. They reduce sleep disruptors such as caffeine and alcohol, and wake up at the same time every day. They engage in regular physical activity (but not close to bedtime), limit naps, manage stress with relaxation techniques, and stay hydrated (while limiting fluids before sleep). They try so hard but, despite doing everything right, they still struggle to fall asleep or stay asleep through the night. This can be exhausting and depressing, especially with the common narrative that ongoing poor sleep can increase the risk of dementia, depression, obesity and diabetes, which only adds to their anxiety. It feels like we can't win.

Options and solutions

Dr Schaedel explains, 'While good sleep hygiene habits are important for making healthy sleep better, they are not an appropriate treatment if you have a sleep disorder, like insomnia. There's never been any evidence that sleep hygiene (on its own) will get your insomnia better. Besides, you are okay if you have not been sleeping well for a prolonged period of time. Humans are naturally built to endure extended periods without sleep. This allows us to adjust to new situations and life events.'

This blew my mind, and I hope many of you who feel the pressure of doing everything to create a healthy sleep hygiene will find it reassuring. You have simply not (yet) embarked on the right treatment to help your insomnia.

With the right treatment, sufferers can recover from insomnia in up to 70 per cent of cases.

Dr Schaedel explains that many of her patients think that their hormone levels alone or the medication, such as tamoxifen or aromatase inhibitors, they have to take are responsible for their poor sleep. And so they might conclude that, unless they stop the medication or get their hormones back, they will also not get their sleep back. 'While cancer or its treatment may trigger sleep issues, they are not necessarily the sole cause of the ongoing problem. It's important to recognise that there is often a distinction between what initially triggers the sleep problem and what keeps it going. Irrespective of the trigger, our brains are always learning and shortcutting and so can easily develop a new habit, which keeps us stuck in a disturbed sleep pattern. The good news is that, due to the neuroplasticity of the brain, you can also relearn and shift your brain back to a healthier space by employing the right evidence-based techniques,' Dr Schaedel explains.

- Before you decide what your next steps will be, be a bit of a detective and try to assess why you are waking up. If it is another symptom, like hot flushes or constantly needing a wee in the middle of the night, it will be best to get these symptoms addressed before you embark on treating the insomnia.

- Multiple international bodies advise that cognitive behavioural therapy for insomnia (CBT-I), a specific, step-by-step treatment programme, has been shown to be the most effective in treating insomnia (for details on this see pages 195–199). CBT-I can be accessed in various ways and there are online versions available free of charge too. Look up the free Sleepio tool and contact charities and your doctor to ask what they have to offer. Sleepstation is another clinically validated sleep improvement programme to combat insomnia. You can find out if Sleepstation is available on the NHS in your area by asking your GP.

- Start addressing sleep issues in the morning: aim to get up at around the same time each morning and get some daylight exposure. If you can, go outside. This signals the body to shut down its melatonin production from the night. Try not to sleep in – and, if possible, stick to the same morning routine.

- During the day, build up and boost your natural drive to sleep. Move your body. Even small chunks of exercise and movement can help. Keep your mealtimes as regular as possible. Make dinner your last meal of the day and avoid snacking. If you graze, your body will think it's still being kept active.

- Have a plan for what you will do when you are awake at night. Often, thoughts seem to be much worse at night than they are during the day. Breathing and visualisation exercises can help the brain and thoughts to slow down. If you can tell sleep is not going to come and you have been awake for roughly 20 minutes already, get out of bed and go to another room. Once you start getting sleep cues, go back to bed and see if sleep comes.

- Take the pressure off. You can't force yourself to sleep. All you can do is set yourself up well enough to sleep.

- Consider not using a clock at night, as constant time-watching can make anxiety around sleep worse.

- Sleeping pills may provide temporary relief but, while they may be useful in certain situations, such as during a crisis, they do not address the underlying sleep problems in the long run.

- Some antidepressants can be helpful for people who struggle with anxiety and have trouble sleeping because of it.

- Melatonin is a natural substance produced by our brain. In the US it is available over the counter; in the UK it is available on prescription for the over-55s for short-term use. Its purpose is not to make you fall asleep; it simply assists us in signalling that it's time to drop off. It's not a sedative and won't instantly make you fall asleep. Sleep experts don't find melatonin a very effective treatment, but many people say it helps them. It may be more helpful for jet lag.

As always, I have learned that our community uses strategies that work for them, even if they are outside the guidance as outlined above. There may be less evidence for their effectiveness, but many women say the following strategies help them doze off or promote better sleep quality.

- Audiobooks
- YouTube guided meditations
- Magnesium before bedtime
- Early dinner, a hot bath (be mindful in case they trigger hot flushes for you) and lavender under the pillow
- No sugary foods before bedtime
- An eye mask
- Acupuncture (see pages 163–165)

Skin Changes

For years I shied away from interviewing people on the podcast about skin. It felt a little vain when we had so many more important things to discuss. But when Dr Mandy Leonhardt published her new book, *What Every Woman Needs to Know About Her Skin and Hair,* I really wanted to talk to her. My skin has changed so much over the last couple of years and I am having a hard time right now trying to like my wrinkles and crow's feet. I tell myself I want to learn to embrace myself the way I am, without fillers and Botox. But I am finding it hard. Dr Leonhardt, who is a GP, menopause expert and nutritionist, says, 'As a woman, whether you've got cancer or not, you can't win. You always lose the game of ageing. If you embark on more invasive treatments like a facelift or fillers or Botox, then it is usually noticeable. You'll get judged. If you do nothing, and you just leave your skin to age naturally you get judged as well.'

The female life cycle is very dynamic. Hormonal changes in our body affect our skin and hair from puberty, to when our hormones change throughout the menstrual cycle every single month, to changes during pregnancy, in the post-pregnancy phase, and then during perimenopause and the menopause. And of course, hormones interplay with each other. Thyroid hormones, cortisol, growth hormones and insulin – many hormones have an impact on skin and hair. In particular, oestrogen plays a vital role for skin health as it aids wound healing and increases the skin's water-holding capacity and moisture levels. Oestrogen stimulates the production of collagen in fibroblasts, and it increases hyaluronic acid levels, which help to keep the skin plump and hydrated. The amount of collagen in the skin starts to reduce slowly from the age of twenty-five, and this breakdown accelerates rapidly with the loss of oestrogen at the onset of menopause, which leads to noticeable skin changes. The skin loses around a third of its collagen during the first five postmenopausal years, after which the decline of collagen continues, but at a slower rate. After menopause the skin often feels drier and the gradual thinning and loss of elasticity leads to more wrinkles.

Options and solutions

Here are Dr Leonhardt's top tips for the basic steps in your skincare routine, to help you figure out what makes sense and where we might be wasting our money.

- Cleansing: Over-cleansing can do more harm than good, stripping away the skin's healthy microbiome and protective barrier. Dr Leonhardt advises against using cleansers in the morning, and says that water alone is enough if you go to bed with a clean face. In the evening, especially if you wear make-up or sunscreen, an oil-based cleanser is better than a water- or gel-based one; studies show that oil-based cleansers effectively remove over 90 per cent of sunscreen and make-up, making them particularly beneficial for dry skin.

- Moisturising: Applying a good moisturiser is essential, but an expensive one isn't necessarily better than a cheaper option. Don't look for miracles in a moisturiser. Moisturisers are exactly what it says on the tin – they're supposed to increase the moisture in your skin, make it feel less tight and make it a little plumper, but this is a very short-lived effect. Most moisturisers will not have a significant anti-wrinkle effect on their own. If you have sensitive skin, choose a fragrance-free moisturiser, as fragrances can irritate the skin.

- Dry skin tip: One of Dr Leonhardt's top tips for very dry skin is to use a thin layer of Vaseline over your moisturiser before bedtime. Vaseline is a very affordable, single-ingredient product that's filtered and purified to a medicinal grade. Clinical trials have shown that it prevents trans-epidermal water loss overnight, which is exactly what you want for maintaining skin hydration. After applying your moisturiser to plump the skin, a thin layer of Vaseline around the eyes or on typically dry areas can help trap moisture. This reduces the significant water loss that happens while we sleep.

- Anti-ageing: If you want a real anti-ageing product, then focus on retinoids. These are a group of chemicals that ultimately convert into retinoic acid, the active form, which can be applied directly to the skin or produced within it. Stronger versions, like tretinoin, are prescription-strength and prescribed by dermatologists. Retinoids are proven to stimulate collagen production, increase skin thickness and reduce the appearance of lines and wrinkles over time. However, it is well documented that some women experience adverse effects such as skin irritation, and stronger formulas can cause side effects like peeling, redness and retinoid dermatitis, so they should be used under medical supervision. To minimise irritation, it's often recommended to start with once-a-week applications. Over-the-counter products typically contain retinol, a milder precursor to retinoic acid.

- Sunscreen: Dr Leonhardt recommends always wearing a sunscreen, even in winter, because harmful UV rays penetrate clouds and are still strong enough to cause skin damage and premature ageing and increase the risk of skin cancer. If you want to choose between mineral and a chemical sunscreen, Dr Leonhardt recommends opting for mineral sunscreens, which are usually based on zinc oxide or titanium dioxide, as they are less likely to cause a skin irritation or reactions in sensitive skin. However, if you don't have sensitive skin, then a chemical sunscreen works equally well. Both chemical and mineral sunscreens work by absorbing UV rays and converting them into heat, with each offering different benefits for skin and the environment.

- Collagen: When I asked Mandy about collagen for our skin's appearance she advised, 'If you choose to use collagen supplements, give them about three months to see any potential benefits, but be aware that the claims made about these products might be exaggerated and they may likely not offer good value for money. Many studies are biased, often funded by the manufacturers, and while there is some evidence that Type II collagen may benefit joint health, the evidence for any benefits from Type I/III collagen for skin and hair is minimal.' (For more on collagen post-cancer treatment, see pages 185–187).

- Holistic skin health: Good sleep is crucial for skin health, often more effective than expensive skincare products, as quality rest refreshes and improves your appearance. Magnesium glycinate can support better sleep, as it helps with relaxation. Additionally, managing stress is important since high cortisol levels can negatively impact skin, so addressing both sleep and stress can significantly benefit your skin from within.

- Eating certain foods can significantly support your skin's appearance by boosting hydration and elasticity and reducing signs of ageing. For example, cocoa powder has been shown to improve skin moisture levels and reduce wrinkles due to its high antioxidant content, so enjoying a hot chocolate or adding cocoa powder to a smoothie can be a delicious way to nourish your skin. Additionally, foods rich in phytonutrients – such as berries, red and purple fruits, and red grapes – are packed with antioxidants like resveratrol, which can help protect the skin from oxidative stress and promote a healthy, youthful complexion. Incorporating these nutrient-dense foods into your diet is an easy and enjoyable way to enhance skin health from the inside out.

Weight Gain

Weight gain is a problem for women in menopause in general. 'Fifty per cent of women gain 1.5kg (3lb) every year of their perimenopause and in total gain 10kg (1 stone 5lb) over their perimenopause with or without a cancer diagnosis. Most of those women tend to gain the weight around their middle,' explains menopause dietician and author Nigel Denby.

Nigel has been helping women in menopause with dietary changes and weight loss for decades and he says, 'Early menopause raises the risk of insulin resistance and Type 2 diabetes, which can contribute to weight gain. Additionally, low levels of oestrogen are associated with a change in body fat distribution towards the centre of the abdomen. Suddenly, weight management methods that worked in your twenties and thirties no longer work during perimenopause and menopause, leading to frustration and a loss of control.'

If you are struggling with your weight when it comes to menopause, there are several other things that may be involved. Your metabolic rate is probably slowing down a little. You might be taking medications that are having an impact on the way your body processes energy. Additionally, no matter how many factors there are in your case, there will also be your own habits within all of this that can play a role. Fatigue and muscle loss from treatment can lead to decreased physical activity, while emotional stress might trigger comfort eating and changed eating habits. In short, weight gain is a multifaceted and complex issue and a common challenge for so many women in our community. One lady wrote, 'Before breast cancer I was already in menopause without any symptoms and still the same size since college. Within four months of starting tamoxifen, I'd gained weight rapidly, and eight months later I couldn't wear anything I owned. I want to cry when I look at my old clothes. Clothes, shoes, underwear, even my rings and watches had to be resized! I'm grateful to be cancer-free right now, but don't recognise or feel like myself at all.'

Many women tell me they are very concerned about their weight gain. Studies suggest that obesity after a cancer diagnosis may be associated with a higher risk of cancer recurrence. We also know weight gain can increase the risk of developing other health issues such as cardiovascular disease, diabetes and hypertension. It can feel depressing and deflating when you try so hard to lose weight and you can't seem to shift it.

Nigel Denby told me that weight loss is difficult but possible. 'Creating sustainable habits takes time and effort. You don't need to make all changes at once; instead, focus on building them gradually over time.' Nigel also acknowledges that, for cancer survivors, weight loss can be particularly challenging due to medications like tamoxifen, which can contribute to weight gain. Additionally, survivors often receive advice to eat anything they want during treatment, which can lead to emotional connections with food. But he assured me that despite these challenges, weight loss is still achievable.

Options and solutions

- Start by writing a detailed food and activity diary for at least three to four days. And be honest. Jot down all meals, snacks and drinks you are consuming and all the ways in which you move. You might be surprised by certain things, like how many snacks you eat, or how little you actually walk on an average day. According to research, the average person consumes a significant portion of their daily calories through snacks, often undoing the benefits of eating healthy meals. Look for regularity. If you eat when you are ravenous, you will eat quickly and you will eat until you are stuffed. What we need to do is eat when we're hungry and eat slowly and mindfully so that we just eat until we're satisfied, not stuffed. That is a really difficult thing to do, but it is the key to being able to eat all the things you love.

- Look at the balance of the food groups on your plate. For more details on what your ideal plate should look like, see pages 247–256. How much are you eating? Nigel explains that one of the things he sees an awful lot of is women who don't eat very much throughout the day, but when they sit down in the evening their meal is huge, and it is often followed by snacks. If weight loss is what you are after, you are going to need to consume fewer calories. 'There is just no smoke and mirrors around that,' Nigel says. There are different ways in which you can create a deficit in calories: you can do it just by eating less, or you can increase your muscle mass and make some changes to your diet at the same time. Building muscle is an excellent way to boost your metabolism and help create a calorie deficit indirectly, because with more muscle tissue your body will burn more calories overall.

- Accept that it's not always going to be easy. Whenever you change anything, there's a degree of discomfort until it starts to feel normal.

- Set a goal that makes sense: Nigel explains, 'The reality is you don't need to get down to being a size eight. If you lose 10 per cent of your starting weight, the benefits to your health go through the roof. It's life-changing what 10 per cent weight loss can do and I always say, let's lose 10 per cent first and then see if you want to lose a bit more.'

Our community shared the following tips:

> *'I stripped it right back to a simple calorie deficit. Tracking calories on the free app My Fitness Pal helped me because I had lost a true sense of what calories were in food and what portion sizes should be. I also started to prioritise protein. Still doing it two years on, 16kg (2 stone 5lb) down. It takes some getting used to. It can be done but it's tough!'*

> *'This is the only thing that has worked for me too. I figured out how many calories I burn on a sedentary day (moving very little) and try to achieve a deficit. Any days I am active is a bonus as the deficit is bigger. I am also using My Fitness Tracker. I'm not denying myself anything at all, I love a biscuit with a cup of tea in the evening, but rather than four biscuits like I used to have, I'll just have one. It's really helped me with making better choices on portion sizes, etc. I've dropped nearly 2kg (4lb 5oz) over just a few weeks.'*

CONCLUSION

My hope in writing this book was that you feel empowered, informed and less alone on your journey through menopause after cancer. Its guidance is not just here to help you manage symptoms; I hope it will help you reclaim your health in many different ways, from the physical to the mental, including your confidence and your joy. There is no perfect way forward, only the path that feels right for you.

Rumi, a thirteenth-century Persian poet and philosopher, whose works have inspired millions including myself, with his profound wisdom, wrote:

'Everything you need, your courage, your love, your compassion, your strength – everything you need is already within you.'

I personally hold on to these words often. And now, as we have journeyed through this book together, I want these words to become your reminder too. That you do indeed, have everything you need, to tackle this next chapter of your healing journey – within you already. I believe in your ability to weather your challenges, and I hope this book has been a starting point, whether it's provided you with knowledge, comfort or encouragement– or all three. It's my deepest wish that you take away from these pages whatever you need in this moment.

I trust that this book will act like a good friend, offering support and insight when you need it most. And know that as an organisation, Menopause and Cancer is here for you every step of the way – please reach out to us and together we'll continue to navigate this journey with hope, courage and determination.

You've got this, and we are here to support you.

Together, we are the changemakers of our generation.

Your voice matters. Your story matters.

By speaking up and sharing your experiences, you can be part of a movement that advances research and improves cancer care.

Together, we can create a future where no one has to navigate menopause after cancer alone.

GLOSSARY

Aromatase inhibitors (AIs)

Before the menopause, oestrogen is mainly produced in the ovaries. After the menopause, the ovaries no longer produce oestrogen, but some oestrogen is still made in body fat. This process involves an enzyme (a type of protein) called aromatase. Aromatase inhibitors stop this enzyme from working. Basically, AIs strip the body of all oestrogen.

ASCO (American Society of Clinical Oncology)

Founded in 1964, the American Society of Clinical Oncology is the world's leading professional organisation for doctors and oncology professionals caring for people with cancer.

BMS (British Menopause Society)

The British Menopause Society is the specialist authority for menopause and post-reproductive health in the UK. The BMS educates, informs and guides healthcare professionals, working in both primary and secondary care, on menopause and all aspects of post-reproductive health.

Chemical menopause

Some cancer treatments, particularly those aimed at hormone-sensitive cancers, involve therapies that block or suppress hormone production. These put you into 'chemical menopause' or give you side effects that mimic those of menopause.

Endocrine therapy

Endocrine therapy involves the use of drugs like tamoxifen, aromatase inhibitors or medications that suppress ovarian function and which may cause you to experience menopause symptoms. These medications are an important part of cancer treatment; they stop the effect of oestrogen on breast cancer cells, doing so in different ways.

GSM (genito-urinary syndrome of menopause)

GSM encompasses a large variety of symptoms that include vaginal dryness, irritation or burning, painful intercourse, itching, vaginal discharge, a reduction in vaginal elasticity, frequent urination, urgency, painful urination and urinary tract infections.

HRT (hormone replacement therapy)

In the UK, we use the term hormone replacement therapy when we talk about hormone therapy to treat menopausal symptoms. In the US and other countries, the terms menopause hormone therapy (MHT) or HT (hormone therapy) are most commonly used. Hormone replacement therapy (HRT) can be either either systemic (see page 323) or local (see page 321), depending on how the hormones are delivered and their intended effect. Systemic hormone therapy and local hormone therapy are two very different things, and it's important that you are clear about each one's role in the body so that you can get the help you need.

Localised hormone replacement therapy

The targeted delivery of hormones to a specific area of the body, typically the vagina or vulva. There is minimal absorption into the bloodstream. This localised treatment addresses the genito-urinary syndrome of menopause (GSM; see opposite).

Mediterranean diet

A style of eating inspired by traditional food practices in Mediterranean coastal regions, including Italy, Greece, Turkey, Spain and France. The Mediterranean diet focuses on a variety of plant-based foods like vegetables, fruits and whole grains, complemented by healthy fats mainly from olive oil, avocados, nuts and seeds. It encourages regular portions of legumes for protein and fibre, as well as moderate amounts of fish, particularly oily fish. Dairy, such as yoghurt and cheese, and poultry are included, while red meat and refined sugars are limited.

Oestrogen

Oestrogen is primarily produced in the ovaries, but some is also produced in our adrenal glands and fat tissue. It plays a crucial role in female sexual development and reproductive function (it regulates the menstrual cycle) but it also has many other vital roles: it maintains bone density; influences skin health and collagen production; affects mood, libido and cognitive function; and plays a role in cardiovascular health.

Oestrogen receptors

Oestrogen interacts with different parts of the body by attaching to specific proteins called oestrogen receptors. These are found all over the body, which is why low oestrogen can cause a wide range of symptoms. There are two main types of receptor and they behave differently depending on where they are. In breast tissue, one type can promote cell growth, while the other may slow it down. Breast cancers are often described as ER-positive (ER+) or ER-negative (ER–), depending on their response to oestrogen.

Premature ovarian insufficiency (POI)

Primary ovarian insufficiency (POI) is a condition in which your ovaries stop working before the age of 40. A common sign of POI is irregular or missed periods.

Progesterone

Progesterone is produced in the ovaries, particularly after ovulation, during the second half of the menstrual cycle. Progesterone is crucial for regulating the menstrual cycle and preparing the uterus lining for pregnancy, and working with oestrogen to promote bone health. It also has a calming effect on the brain, which for some women can help improve sleep quality, regulate mood swings and reduce feelings of anxiety.

Pro-inflammatory markers

Pro-inflammatory markers are substances in the blood that indicate inflammation.

Randomised controlled trial (RCT)

A scientific experiment that compares the effectiveness of treatments, drugs or other interventions. A number of similar people are randomly assigned to two or more groups. One group or groups receives a new treatment, while a control group receives either the current standard treatment or a placebo. RCTs are considered the most reliable way to compare treatments.

Surgical menopause

Procedures such as a hysterectomy in which your womb *and* ovaries were also removed, or a bilateral oophorectomy, the surgical removal of both functioning ovaries, can abruptly stop oestrogen and progesterone production. As these hormones play a central role in regulating the menstrual cycles, their sudden absence results in the immediate onset of permanent menopause.

Systemic hormone replacement therapy (HRT)

The administration of hormones, typically oestrogen, progesterone and testosterone, which are absorbed into the bloodstream and circulate throughout the body.

Tamoxifen

Tamoxifen is used to treat oestrogen receptor-positive (ER+) breast cancer and belongs to a class of drugs called selective oestrogen receptor modulators (SERMs). It works by blocking the effects of oestrogen on ER+ breast cancer cells. Tamoxifen doesn't cause menopause, but it can trigger symptoms commonly associated with it. It is used to treat breast cancer in both premenopausal and postmenopausal women.

Testosterone

Testosterone is often thought of as a 'male hormone', but it is also an important female hormone, produced in the ovaries and our adrenal glands. It helps regulate sexual desire, supports muscle mass and helps maintain strong bones.

Vaginal laser

Vaginal laser therapy has emerged as a promising option for managing symptoms of vaginal atrophy and dryness. A probe with a laser is inserted into the vagina; it penetrates the tissue and causes heat-related injury. As the injury heals, collagen production is triggered.

Vaginal moisturiser

Moisturisers and lubricants that do not contain oestrogen but act to keep the tissues well hydrated and feeling less sore. Moisturisers are for help throughout the day and are longer-lasting, so you might only need to use a moisturiser every two or three days.

Vaginal oestrogen

Vaginal oestrogen is a topical, local oestrogen therapy used to treat the genito-urinary syndrome of menopause (GSM). GSM results from a decline in oestrogen levels and encompasses a large variety of symptoms that include vaginal dryness, irritation or burning, painful intercourse, itching, vaginal discharge, a reduction in vaginal elasticity, frequent urination, urgency, painful urination and urinary tract infections.

FURTHER SUPPORT AND RESOURCES

I invite you to visit our website: menopauseandcancer.org. There, you'll find a wealth of additional support, including a video library, helpful articles and details about our workshops and events. You will also be able to join the online community.

Remember to download the digital handbook, which includes links to many other organisations and charities, and includes helpful tips and resources, and even studies you can share with your doctors. Simply scan the QR code below – leave your email and we'll send the handbook straight to your inbox.

You can also get a copy by visiting:

www.menopauseandcancer.org/book

PLEASE LEAVE A REVIEW

Spreading the word about this book helps more and more cancer survivors access support and guidance. If you can leave a review on the platform on which you bought this book, it will help others find and access its information. Thank you!

ACKNOWLEDGEMENTS

I would like to thank all the women in my community whom I have walked with, laughed with, cried with, shared stories with, and hugged, for allowing me to see them for who they are. It is this deep connection to humanity and life itself, but also their tangible need for this book, that kept me going when the writing process was tough.

To all the incredible doctors and experts who have helped shape this book and who offer their help in our day-to-day work at Menopause and Cancer – thank you. You are changemakers, leading forces in your fields, and your passion for providing your patients with the right support will have a huge ripple effect across the world – I know it.

To my editor, Imogen Fortes – thank you. You took me on as a rogue client. I had no publishing deal, no agent, just documents and documents filled with passion, and without your meticulous help and experience – but also your belief that our community needs this book – I would not have been able to push this over the finish line. Our work together has taken us across the UK, Austria and France, and what a journey it has been! On behalf of all of us – thank you for believing in us.

To my daughters, I kept telling you multiple times, 'That's it. I'm done. I can't do it.' You are the forces of the next generation – and I am so proud of each of you. You show up in life in your many different brilliant ways and together, we have learned through our ups and downs that we can do hard things, and that it's always, always worth it to keep going. Thank you for your many 'You can do it, Mum, I am proud of you' moments.

To my husband, where do I even begin? Thank you for your unwavering support in everything I do, from selling cute boots (you know what I mean) to taking endless pictures of me in yoga poses all across the world. Without your endless encouragement for all of my passions and projects, we would not have a not-for-profit organisation or this book. Your expansive thinking and daily graft have allowed me to grow and believe that I can do this.

To Laura, who joined our first Menopause and Cancer wellbeing retreat and casually mentioned, just before we all left, that she is a book designer. From that moment, there was no looking back! Laura, you are the most incredible human – I fell in love with every cover you designed. At that moment, this truly became a book from the community, for the community. Thank you.

And last but not least, thank you to the wise woman I am so grateful to call my mum. You have taught me more than I can ever put into words, but, most importantly, you gave me the love and wings I needed to fly, and because of you I truly understand, 'in the end, love remains, and that's all that matters.'

WITH GRATITUDE TO OUR MEDICAL CONTRIBUTORS

I feel incredibly fortunate to have had the support, expertise, and encouragement of so many professionals while writing this book. From oncologists and menopause specialists to nutritionists, dietitians, researchers, and exercise experts – each one brought something valuable to the table, and their contributions helped shape this into the holistic, practical guide I hoped it would be.

I want to thank, in particular, Mr Vikram Talaulikar and Dr Alison Macbeth. Their generosity, time and unwavering support have meant the world to me. They didn't just help shape these pages – they helped shape the impact I hope this book will have on anyone navigating life after cancer.

Thank you for walking this path with me.

Expert Contributors:

Dr Laila Agrawal – *Medical oncologist and haematologist, breast cancer specialist (US)*

Professor Sarah Berry – *Department of Nutritional Sciences, King's College London & ZOE Chief Scientist*

Barbie Boules – *Dietician (US)*

Professor Anna Campbell – *Professor of Clinical Exercise Science, founder of CanRehab Trust*

Nigel Denby – *Dietician with special interest in menopause*

Sam Evans – *Sexual health educator, founder of adult toy business Jo Divine*

Dr Nina Fuller-Shavel – *Integrative medicine doctor (UK)*

Dr Rebecca Glaser – *Breast cancer surgeon (US)*

Dr Melanie Hacking – *GP, BMS Menopause Specialist*

Dr Susanne Hooper – *GP, BMS Menopause Specialist*

Dr Olivia Hum – *GP, BMS Menopause Specialist*

Dr Shelly Latte-Naor – *Integrative medicine doctor, Memorial Sloan Kettering (US)*

Dr Mandy Leonhardt – *GP, BMS Menopause Specialist, nutritionist*

Professor Claire Macaulay – *Breast oncologist, Beatson West of Scotland Cancer Centre*

Dr Alison Macbeth – *GP, BMS Menopause Specialist, breast speciality doctor*

Melinda McDougall – *Medical herbalist specialising in menopause*

Dr Corinne Menn – *OBGYN and Menopause Society Certified Practitioner (US)*

Sarah Newman – *Cancer exercise specialist*

Kate Pleace – *Fertility and menopause specialist nurse*

Rebekah Rotstein – *Founder of Buff Bones®, exercise specialist*

Dr Zoe Schaedel – *GP, BMS Menopause Specialist, sleep expert*

Professor Richard Simcock – *Consultant clinical oncologist (UK), CMO MacMillan*

Mr Vikram Talaulikar – *Reproductive medicine specialist, BMS Menopause Specialist*

Dr Eleonora Teplinsky – *Medical oncologist (US), breast & gynaecological cancers*

Dr Lindsey Thomas – *GP, BMS Menopause Specialist*

Andrea Ward – *Team leader, breast care nurse team, York & Scarborough NHS Trust*

Julie Webb – *Registered nutritional therapist*

Lavinia Winch – *Sexual health educator, YES ambassador*

Hillary Wright – *Registered dietitian (US)*

Dr Angela Wright – *Psychosexual therapist, BMS Menopause Specialist*

ABOUT THE AUTHOR

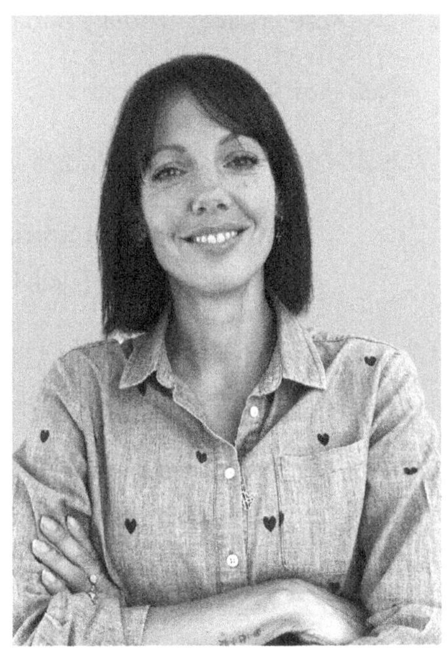

Dani Binnington is the founder of Menopause and Cancer, the world's only not-for-profit organisation dedicated to supporting cancer survivors navigating treatment-induced menopause. As a breast cancer survivor herself, Dani's personal experience with surgical menopause after cancer inspired her mission to create a global conversation around survivorship, holistic wellbeing and inclusive menopause care.

With a background as a fashion jewellery designer, Dani retrained as a yoga teacher and, while working as a wellbeing expert, created a Facebook community to connect with other cancer survivors facing the same menopause struggles. This was the beginning of a journey that has seen her curate workshops, programmes and initiatives recognised for their positive impact on survivors worldwide.

In 2022, Dani launched The Menopause and Cancer Podcast, which has become an invaluable resource for survivors and healthcare professionals alike. She interviews leading medical experts and shares survivor stories, offering evidence-based guidance and practical tools – 'with heaps of compassion,' as her audience says.

Dani's work has been featured on UK television, including *This Morning,* as well as in the national press. She continues to be a sought-after speaker, writer and educator on the unique challenges of menopause after cancer.

Through her book, community work and ongoing advocacy, Dani is committed to ensuring no one feels alone in their survivorship journey. Her mission is to empower, educate and inspire others to know that there is always something they can do to try to feel better.

Dani lives in the UK with her husband and three daughters, where she dedicates her life to creating change. One conversation at a time.

ENDNOTES

Introduction

1 https://www.breastcancer.org/treatment-side-effects/menopause

2 https://www.thelancet.com/journals/lancet/article/PIIS0140-6736(23)02802-7/fulltext

Chapter 1:

3 https://www.thelancet.com/journals/lancet/article/PIIS0140-6736(23)02802-7/fulltext

4 https://www.macmillan.org.uk/cancer-information-and-support/impacts-of-cancer/menopausal-symptoms-and-cancer-treatment

5 https://www.sciencedirect.com/science/article/pii/S2451965020301447

6 https://www.cancerresearchuk.org/about-cancer/coping/physically/sex/women/menopausal-symptoms

7 https://pubmed.ncbi.nlm.nih.gov/39999470

Chapter 2:

8 https://bssm.org.uk/wp-content/uploads/2024/03/BSSM-Position-statement-for-management-of-genitourinary-syndrome-of-the-menopause-GSM.pdf

9 https://bssm.org.uk/wp-content/uploads/2024/03/BSSM-Position-statement-for-management-of-genitourinary-syndrome-of-the-menopause-GSM.pdf

10 https://pmc.ncbi.nlm.nih.gov/articles/PMC8894268

Chapter 3:

11 https://www.nhs.uk/conditions/early-menopause

12 https://thebms.org.uk/menopause-specialists/overview

Chapter 4:

13 https://www.nice.org.uk/news/articles/discussion-aid-to-support-clinical-conversations-about-hrt-published-alongside-updated-guidance

14 https://menopause.org/wp-content/uploads/professional/2023-nonhormone-therapy-position-statement.pdf

15 The Complete Guide to the Menopause, Dr Annice Mukherjee, p.122.

Chapter 5:

16 https://menopause.org/wp-content/uploads/professional/2023-nonhormone-therapy-position-statement.pdf

17 https://thebms.org.uk/wp-content/uploads/2022/12/02-BMS-TfC-Prescribable-alternatives-to-HRT-NOV2022-A.pdf, accessed 10 October 2024.

18 https://thebms.org.uk/wp-content/uploads/2024/06/04-BMS-ConsensusStatement-Non-hormonal-based-treatments-JUNE2024-B.pdf, accessed 10 October 2024.

19 https://thebms.org.uk/wp-content/uploads/2022/12/02-BMS-TfC-Prescribable-alternatives-to-HRT-NOV2022-A.pdf, accessed 10 October 24.

20 https://www.yesyesyes.org/pages/yes-the-nhs-faq

21 https://www.nice.org.uk/guidance/IPG697/chapter/1-Recommendations

22 https://menopause.org/wp-content/uploads/professional/2023-nonhormone-therapy-position-statement.pdf

23 https://thebms.org.uk/wp-content/uploads/2022/12/02-BMS-TfC-Prescribable-alternatives-to-HRT-NOV2022-A.pdf

Chapter 6:

NB note 4 in its entirety refers to the table 'Recommendations for the use of hormone replacement therapy by cancer type' on p00.

24 https://thebms.org.uk/wp-content/uploads/2023/10/02-BMS-ConsensusStatement-BMS-WHC-2020-Recommendations-on-HRT-in-menopausal-women-SEPT2023-A.pdf, accessed 11 October 2024.

25 The 'ELITE-HRT' study (Early versus Late Intervention Trial with Estradiol-Hormone Replacement Therapy) was launched to re-examine the findings of the Women's Health Initiative (WHI) and investigate the risks and benefits of hormone replacement therapy (HRT) in postmenopausal women.

26 https://thebms.org.uk/publications/consensus-statements/bms-whcs-2020-recommendations-on-hormone-replacement-therapy-in-menopausal-women

27 NB this note in its entirety refers to the table 'Recommendations for the use of hormone replacement therapy by cancer type' on p00.

28 [1] Abubakar, M., Chang-Claude, J., Ali, H.R. et al. Etiology of hormone receptor positive breast cancer differs by levels of histologic grade and proliferation. Int J Cancer. 2018;143(4):746–757.[2] Ellingjord-Dale M., Vos, L., Tretli, S. et al. Parity, hormones and breast cancer subtypes – results from a large nested case-control study in a national screening program. Breast Cancer Res. 2017;19(1):10. [3] Salagame, U., Banks, E., O'Connell D.L. et al. Menopausal hormone therapy use and breast cancer risk by receptor subtypes: results from the New South Wales Cancer Lifestyle and Evaluation of Risk (CLEAR) study. PLoS One. 2018;13(11):e0205034.[4] Sisti, J.S., Collins, L.C., Beck, A.H. et al. Reproductive risk factors in relation to molecular subtypes of breast cancer: results from the nurses' health studies. Int J Cancer. 2016;138(10):2346–2356.[5] Anderson, K.N., Schwab, R.B., Martinez, M.E. Reproductive risk factors and breast cancer subtypes: a review of the literature. Breast Cancer Res Treat. 2014;144(1):1 – 10.[6] Morra, A., Jung, A.Y., Behrens, S. et al. Breast cancer risk factors and survival by tumor subtype: pooled analyses from the breast cancer association consortium. Cancer Epidemiol Biomark Prev PublAm Assoc Cancer Res Cosponsored Am Soc Prev Oncol. 2021;30(4):623–642.[7] Chlebowski, R.T., Anderson, G.L., Aragaki, A.K. et al. Association of menopausal hormone therapy with breast cancer incidence and mortality during long-term follow-up of the women's health initiative randomized clinical trials. JAMA. 2020;324(4):369–380.[8] Santen, R.J., Stuenkel, C.A., Davis S.R. et al. Managing menopausal symptoms and associated clinical issues in breast cancer survivors. J Clin Endocrinol Metab. 2017;102(10):3647–3661.

Marsden, J., Whitehead, M., A'Hern, R. et al. Are randomized trials of hormone replacement therapy in symptomatic women with breast cancer feasible? Fertil Steril. 2000;73(2):292–299.[20] Kenemans, P., Bundred, N.J., Foidart, J.M. et al. Safety and efficacy of tibolone in breast-cancer patients with vasomotor symptoms: a double-blind, randomised, non-inferiority trial. Lancet Oncol.2009; 10(2): 135–146.[21] Kloosterboer, H.J. Tibolone: a steroid with a tissue-specific mode of action. J Steroid Biochem Mol Biol. 2001;76(1–5):231–238.[22] Poggio, F., Del Mastro, L., Bruzzone, M. et al. Safety of systemic hormone replacement therapy in breast cancer survivors: a systematic review and meta-analysis. Breast Cancer Res Treat. 2022; 191(2):269–275.[23] Ugras, S.K., Layeequr Rahman, R. Hormone replacement therapy after breast cancer: yes, no or maybe? Mol Cell Endocrinol. 2021;525: 111180.[24] Mruthyunjayappa, S., Zhang, K., Zhang, L. et al. Synchronous and metachronous bilateral breast cancer: clinicopathologic characteristics and prognostic outcomes. Hum Pathol. 2019;92: 1–9.[25] van Barele, M., Heemskerk-Gerritsen, B.A.M., Louwers, Y.V. et al.Estrogens and progestogens in triple negative breast cancer: do they harm? Cancers. 2021; 13(11):2506.[26] The 2022 Hormone Therapy Position Statement of The North American Menopause Society Advisory Panel. The 2022 hormone therapy position statement of The North American Menopause Society. Menopause N Y N. 2022;29(7):76794.[27] Mendoza, N., Ramírez, I., de la Viuda, E. et al. Eligibility criteria for Menopausal Hormone Therapy (MHT): a position statement from a consortium of scientific societies for the use of MHT in women with medical conditions. MHT Eligibility Criteria Group. Maturitas.2022; 166:65–85.[28] Shufelt, C., Bairey Merz, C.N., Pettinger, M.B. et al. Estrogen-alone therapy and invasive breast cancer incidence by dose, formulation, and route of delivery: findings from the WHI observational study. Menopause. 2018;25(9):985–991.[29] Bhupathiraju, S.N., Grodstein, F., Stampfer, M.J. et al. Vaginal estrogen use and chronic disease risk in the Nurses' Health Study. Menopause N Y N. 2019;26(6):603–610.[30] Lyytinen, H., Pukkala, E., Ylikorkala, O. Breast cancer risk in postmenopausal women using estrogen-only therapy. Obstet Gynecol.2006; 108(6): 1354–1360.[31] Faubion, S.S., Larkin, L.C., Stuenkel, C.A. et al. Management of genitourinary syndrome of menopause in women with or at high risk for breast cancer: consensus recommendations from The North American Menopause Society and The International Society for the Study of Women's Sexual Health. Menopause. 2018;25(6):596–608.[32] Rees, M., Angioli, R., Coleman, R.L. et al. European Menopause and Andropause Society (EMAS) and International Gynecologic Cancer Society (IGCS) position statement on managing the menopause after gynecological cancer: focus on menopausal symptoms and osteoporosis. Maturitas. 2020; 134:56–61.[33] Paluch-Shimon, S., Cardoso, F., Partridge, A.H. et al. ESO-ESMO 4thinternational consensus guidelines for breast cancer in young women (BCY4). Ann Oncol. 2020;31(6):674–696.[34] Cold, S., Cold, F., Jensen, M.B. et al. Systemic or vaginal hormone therapy After early breast cancer: a Danish observational cohort study. J Natl Cancer Inst. 2022; 114(10): 1347–1354. [35] Barton, D.L., Shuster, L.T., Dockter, T. et al. Systemic and local effects of vaginal dehydroepiandrosterone (DHEA): NCCTG N10C1 (alliance). Support Care Cancer. 2018;26(4):1335–1343.[36] Gernier, F., Ahmed-Lecheheb, D., Pautier, P. et al. Chronic fatigue, quality of life and long-term side-effects of chemotherapy inpatients treated for non-epithelial ovarian cancer: national case control protocol study of the GINECO-Vivrovaire rare tumors INCaFrench network for rare malignant ovarian tumors. BMC Cancer.2021;21(1):1147.[37] Gernier, F., Gompel, A., Rousset-Jablonski, C. et al. Menopausal symptoms in epithelial ovarian cancer survivors: a GINECOVIVROVAIRE2 study. Gynecol Oncol. 2021;163(3):598–604. [38] Rousset-Jablonski, C., Selle, F., Adda-Herzog, E. et al. Fertility preservation, contraception and menopause hormone therapy in women treated for rare ovarian tumours: guidelines from the French national network dedicated to rare gynaecological cancers. Eur J Cancer Oxf Engl 1990. 2019;116:35–44.[39] Guidozzi, F. & Daponte, A. Estrogen replacement therapy for ovarian carcinoma survivors: a randomized controlled trial. Cancer. 1999;86(6):1013–1018.[40] Li, L., Pan, Z., Gao, K. et al. Impact of post-operative hormone replacement therapy on life quality and prognosis in patients with ovarian malignancy. Oncol Lett. 2012;3(1):244–249.[41] Eeles, R.A., Morden, J.P., Gore, M. et al. Adjuvant hormone therapy may improve survival in epithelial ovarian cancer: results of the AHT randomized trial. J Clin Oncol. 2015;33(35):4138–4144.[42] Li, D., Ding, C.Y., Qiu, L.H. Postoperative hormone replacement therapy for epithelial ovarian cancer patients: a systematic review and meta-analysis. Gynecol Oncol. 2015;139(2):355–362. [43] Sinno, A.K., Pinkerton, J., Febbraro, T. et al. Hormone therapy (HT) in women with gynecologic cancers and in women at high risk for developing a gynecologic cancer: a Society of Gynecologic Oncology (SGO) clinical practice statement: this practice statement has been endorsed by The North American Menopause Society. Gynecol Oncol. 2020;157(2):303–306.[44] Barakat, R.R., Bundy, B.N., Spirtos, N.M. et al. Randomized double blind trial of estrogen replacement therapy versus placebo in stage I or II endometrial cancer: a Gynecologic Oncology Group Study. J Clin Oncol. 2006;24(4):587–592.[45] Maxwell, G.L., Tian, C., Risinger, J.I. et al. Racial disparities in recurrence among patients with early-stage endometrial cancer: is recurrence increased in black patients who receive estrogen replacement therapy? Cancer. 2008;113(6):1431–1437.[46] Edey, K.A., Rundle, S., Hickey, M. Hormone replacement therapy for women previously treated for endometrial cancer. Cochrane Database Syst Rev. 2018;5(5):CD008830.

British Gynaecological Cancer Society and British Menopause Society guidelines, accessed 2 December 2024.

29 https://www.nice.org.uk/guidance/ng101/chapter/Recommendations#complications-of-local-treatment-and-menopausal-symptoms

30 https://menopause.org/wp-content/uploads/professional/nams-2022-hormone-therapy-position-statement.pdf

31 https://lizearlewellbeing.com/healthy-living/breast-cancer-hrt-kirsty-lang

32 https://www.thelancet.com/journals/lancet/article/PIIS0140-6736(04)15493-7/abstract

33 https://academic.oup.com/jnci/article-abstract/97/7/533/2544226?redirectedFrom=fulltext, accessed 11 October 2024.

34 https://pubmed.ncbi.nlm.nih.gov/34731351

35 https://pubmed.ncbi.nlm.nih.gov/29763858

36 https://pmc.ncbi.nlm.nih.gov/articles/PMC8196589

37 https://ascopubs.org/doi/10.1200/EDBK_100032

38 https://ascopost.com/issues/december-25-2020/sexual-health-an-issue-for-many-survivors-of-cancer

39 https://bmjmedicine.bmj.com/content/bmjmed/3/1/e000753.full.pdf

40 https://bssm.org.uk/wp-content/uploads/2023/02/GSM-BSSM.pdf

41 https://pubmed.ncbi.nlm.nih.gov/37383954

42 https://pubmed.ncbi.nlm.nih.gov/35854422

43 https://pmc.ncbi.nlm.nih.gov/articles/PMC9905959

44 https://jamanetwork.com/journals/jamaoncology/article-abstract/2811413

45 https://www.ajog.org/article/S0002-9378(24)01126-8/abstract?fbclid=PAZXh0bgNhZW0CMTEAAaahp T8hBm4WxWMPXzKZcKgie3unJHcDAcfKOzL 9PxA1cHiaBf-tj4qsc_aem_qpFn2VYdwpTLStLOfDchqA

46 https://journals.sagepub.com/doi/full/10.1177/20533691231208473

Chapter 7:

47 https://www.webmd.com/breast-cancer/breast-cancer-types-er-positive-her2-positive

48 https://www.macmillan.org.uk/cancer-information-and-support/treatments-and-drugs/hormonal-therapy-for-breast-cancer

49 https://pmc.ncbi.nlm.nih.gov/articles/PMC9073292

50 https://www.sciencedirect.com/science/article/pii/S0960977622000121

51 https://www.who.int/news-room/fact-sheets/detail/breast-cancer

52 https://thebms.org.uk/wp-content/uploads/2022/12/02-BMS-TfC-Prescribable-alternatives-to-HRT-NOV2022-A.pdf

53 https://owise.uk/tamoxifen-what-you-should-avoid

54 https://www.ncbi.nlm.nih.gov/pmc/articles/PMC10558019/#:~:text=Alcohol%20should%20be%20avoided%20or%20limited%20while%20taking%20aromatase%20inhibitors,with%20the%20efficacy%20of%20exemestane

55 https://pmc.ncbi.nlm.nih.gov/articles/PMC10558019/#:~:text=Alcohol%20should%20be%20avoided%20or%20limited%20while%20taking%20aromatase%20inhibitors,with%20the%20efficacy%20of%20exemestane

Chapter 8:

56 https://www.cancerresearchuk.org/about-cancer/treatment/complementary-alternative-therapies/research/about#:~:text=Researchers%20estimate%20that%2030%20to,with%20cancer%20view%20complementary%20therapies

57 https://ascopubs.org/doi/full/10.1200/JCO.22.01357#tbl3

58 https://jamanetwork.com/journals/jamanetworkopen/fullarticle/2798317

59 https://www.medpagetoday.com/hematologyoncology/breastcancer/110797?th=1&utm_source=facebook&utm_medium=cpc&utm_campaign=fb-md-cbtm-onc-pibr&trw=no&scrf=1&xid=fb-md-cbtm-onc-pibr&utm_id=6498678796877&utm_content=6555872053877&utm_term=6498678797477&fbclid=IwY2xjawFZEcxleHRuA2FlbQIxMQABHeGkd5spos3p-rZn0I1uLfH_8yNhO3yjLlg8nz-1PnezAGergmXcVuNUpg_aem_vf6-VJaePK7gX1zUTIGErA

60 https://www.nhs.uk/conditions/herbal-medicines

61 https://mpowder.store/pages/cancer-and-menopause

62 https://clinicaltrials.gov/study/NCT05664477

63 https://tucson.com/news/local/subscriber/tucson-medical-startup-university-of-arizona/article_0d422df8-7e94-11ee-b63f-f75185114024.html

64 https://www.neutherapeutics.com/about

65 https://pubmed.ncbi.nlm.nih.gov/26455645/#:~:text=Results%25253A%252520A%252520statistically%252520significant%252520

66 https://www.mskcc.org/cancer-care/integrative-medicine/herbs/black-cohosh

67 https://www.sciencedirect.com/science/article/abs/pii/S0960076013000381?via%3Dihub

68 https://www.tandfonline.com/doi/full/10.1080/13697137.2020.1820477

69 https://www.tandfonline.com/doi/full/10.3109/09513590.2010.538097

70 https://www.mskcc.org/cancer-care/integrative-medicine/herbs/st-john-wort

71 https://www.mskcc.org/cancer-care/integrative-medicine/herbs/ashwagandha

72 https://cdn.shopify.com/s/files/1/0400/9892/2660/files/MPowder_Naturopathy_Menopause.pdf?v=1706803855

73 https://pubmed.ncbi.nlm.nih.gov/23142798

74 https://mpowder.store/pages/cancer-and-menopause

75 https://www.sciencedirect.com/science/article/abs/pii/S0002916523663427?via%3Dihub

76 https://www.massgeneralbrigham.org/en/about/newsroom/press-releases/multivitamins-improve-memory-and-slow-cognitive-aging

77 https://www.nhs.uk/conditions/vitamins-and-minerals/vitamin-d

78 https://pmc.ncbi.nlm.nih.gov/articles/PMC3440651/#:~:text=treatment%20of%20cancer.-,Vitamin%20D%20deficiency%20has%20been%20found%20to%20be%20associated%20with,it%20a%20potential%20risk%20factor

79 https://theros.org.uk/information-and-support/bone-health/nutrition-for-bones/calcium/?_gl=1*ms5rok*_up*MQ..&gclid=CjwKCAjwxY-3BhAuEiwAu7Y6sziQX-J-mHN9x1Yzg6eToW3SxMQ0AbyjclaKss6Qqm_osTuwswHBahoCvCgQAvD_BwE

80 https://ods.od.nih.gov/factsheets/Magnesium-HealthProfessional

81 https://www.health.harvard.edu/staying-healthy/turmeric-benefits-a-look-at-the-evidence

82 https://www.health.harvard.edu/staying-healthy/turmeric-benefits-a-look-at-the-evidence

83 https://cdn.shopify.com/s/files/1/0400/9892/2660/files/MPOWDER_Naturopathy_Menopause_c875c653-27e7-42b2-a5e4-a38335905ce2.pdf?v=1740511800

84 https://www.womens-health-concern.org/wp-content/uploads/2023/02/02-WHC-FACTSHEET-CBT-WOMEN-FEB-2023-A.pdf

85 https://thebms.org.uk/wp-content/uploads/2022/12/01-BMS-TfC-CBT-NOV2022-A.pdf

86 https://academic.oup.com/jncics/article/8/3/pkae041/7680549?utm_source=chatgpt.com&login=false

87 https://www.england.nhs.uk/mental-health/adults/nhs-talking-therapies

88 https://pubmed.ncbi.nlm.nih.gov/38426042

89 https://pmc.ncbi.nlm.nih.gov/articles/PMC9990873

90 https://ascopubs.org/doi/10.1200/JCO.2023.41.16_suppl.12111

91 https://pubmed.ncbi.nlm.nih.gov/28917368

92 https://www.sciencedirect.com/science/article/pii/S0272735824001260

93 https://ascopubs.org/doi/10.1200/JCO.2015.65.7874

94 https://www.occupationaltherapy.com/ot-ceus/course/journaling-in-ot-to-address-5580

95 https://pmc.ncbi.nlm.nih.gov/articles/PMC3927735

96 https://positivepsychology.com/benefits-of-gratitude

97 https://pubmed.ncbi.nlm.nih.gov/26166171

Chapter 9:

98 'American College of Sports Medicine Roundtable Report on Physical Activity, Sedentary Behavior, and Cancer Prevention and Control'; Patel, Alpa V., Friedenreich, Christine M., Moore, Steven C., Hayes, Sandra C., Silver, Julie K., Campbell, Kristin L., Winters-Stone, Kerri, Gerber, Lynn H., George, Stephanie M., Fulton, Janet E., Denlinger, Crystal, Stephen Morris, G., Hue, Trisha, Schmitz, Kathryn H., Matthews, Charles E.; Medicine and Science in Sports and Exercise, 2019

99 https://www.cosa.org.au/media/332488/cosa-position-statement-v4-web-final.pdf

100 https://acsm.org/physical-activity-guidelines-cancer-infographic

101 https://jamanetwork.com/journals/jamaoncology/article-abstract/2817661

102 https://pubmed.ncbi.nlm.nih.gov/31617590

103 https://acsm.org/physical-activity-guidelines-cancer-infographic

104 https://journals.lww.com/acsm-msse/Fulltext/2019/11000/Exercise_Guidelines_for_Cancer_Survivors_.23.aspx

105 https://research-repository.griffith.edu.au/items/f1087d47-09ba-4cd7-b3b3-f53d6c5c8677

106 https://www.exerciseismedicine.org/wp-content/uploads/2023/04/MTC-brochure-DIGITAL-update.pdf

107 https://acsjournals.onlinelibrary.wiley.com/doi/full/10.3322/caac.21721

108 https://pubmed.ncbi.nlm.nih.gov/28253393

109 https://acsm.org/physical-activity-guidelines-cancer-infographic

110 https://acsm.org/physical-activity-guidelines-cancer-infographic

111 https://acsm.org/physical-activity-guidelines-cancer-infographic

112 https://pmc.ncbi.nlm.nih.gov/articles/PMC10095144/#:~:text=The%20characteristic%20of%20premature%20and,osteoporosis%2C%20depression%2C%20and%20parkinsonism

Chapter 10:

113 https://www.frontiersin.org/journals/endocrinology/articles/10.3389/fendo.2022.886824/full

114 https://www.nia.nih.gov/news/mind-and-mediterranean-diets-linked-fewer-signs-alzheimers-brain-pathology

115 https://pubmed.ncbi.nlm.nih.gov/23553160

116 https://www.bda.uk.com/resource/fibre.html

117 https://www.bhf.org.uk/informationsupport/heart-matters-magazine/nutrition/fibre

118 https://assets.publishing.service.gov.uk/media/5a749fece5274a44083b82d8/government_dietary_recommendations.pdf

119 https://www.mdpi.com/2076-3921/12/2/470

120 https://www.mdpi.com/1424-8247/17/6/692

121 https://nutritionsource.hsph.harvard.edu/healthy-eating-plate

122 https://www.wcrf.org/living-well/living-with-cancer/your-questions-answered/how-important-is-protein-during-cancer

123 https://www.aicr.org/cancer-prevention/how-to-prevent-cancer

124 https://www.aicr.org/cancer-prevention/how-to-prevent-cancer

125 Reference The Complete Guide book

126 Book details + page ref

127 https://owise.uk/tamoxifen-what-you-should-avoid

128 https://pmc.ncbi.nlm.nih.gov/articles/PMC5540319/#:~:text=The%20current%20data%20suggest%20that,associated%20with%20obesity%20and%20inflammation

129 https://www.wcrf.org/wp-content/uploads/2024/11/Policy-position-alcohol-cancer-risk-0924.pdf

130 https://www.thelancet.com/journals/ebiom/article/PIIS2352-3964(22)00485-6/fulltext

131 https://zoe.com/learn/gut-microbiome-menopause-changes

Chapter 11:

132 https://www.nhs.uk/mental-health/talking-therapies-medicine-treatments/talking-therapies-and-counselling/cognitive-behavioural-therapy-cbt/overview

133 https://ascopubs.org/doi/10.1200/JCO.23.00857

134 https://www.rcot.co.uk/learn-about-occupational-therapy/ot-advice/lift-up/energy

135 https://owise.uk/hot-flushes-causes-management

136 https://pubmed.ncbi.nlm.nih.gov/17476146/#:~:text=Women%20with%20an%20early%20menopause,appropriate%20anti%2Dresorptive%20therapy%20initiated

137 https://theros.org.uk/risk-checker?gad_source=1&gclid=CjwKCAjw68K4BhAuEiwAylp3kvEzHj84xAdLIVQtDVPSbHVDhsdYH0VpGXSnc_L3PjqC2TaucouxvRoCkgsQAvD_BwE&campaign=77a866ee-c708-ed11-82e5-0022481b5a28

138 https://theros.org.uk/blog/2021-03-22-what-s-the-menopause-got-to-do-with-bone-health/#:~:text=If%20you%20have%20an%20early,weaker%20bones%20in%20later%20life

139 https://theros.org.uk/media/0o5h1153/ros-strong-steady-straight-quick-guide-february-2019.pdf

INDEX

Made in the USA
Monee, IL
17 July 2025

21340424R00218